Nutrition and Fitness: Mental Health

Nutrition and Fitness: Mental Health

Editor

Riccardo Dalle Grave

MDPI • Basel • Beijing • Wuhan • Barcelona • Belgrade • Manchester • Tokyo • Cluj • Tianjin

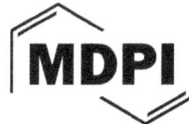

Editor
Riccardo Dalle Grave
Villa Garda Hospital
Italy

Editorial Office
MDPI
St. Alban-Anlage 66
4052 Basel, Switzerland

This is a reprint of articles from the Special Issue published online in the open access journal *Nutrients* (ISSN 2072-6643) (available at: https://www.mdpi.com/journal/nutrients/special_issues/nutrition_mental).

For citation purposes, cite each article independently as indicated on the article page online and as indicated below:

LastName, A.A.; LastName, B.B.; LastName, C.C. Article Title. *Journal Name* **Year**, *Article Number*, Page Range.

ISBN 978-3-03943-112-0 (Hbk)
ISBN 978-3-03943-113-7 (PDF)

Contents

About the Editor

Riccardo Dalle Grave, MD. Director of the Department of Eating and Weight Disorders at Villa Garda Hospital (Garda, VR, Italy). In this department, he developed an original treatment for eating disorders, based entirely on enhanced cognitive behavior therapy (CBT-E), adaptation of outpatient CBT-E for adolescents with eating disorders, and personalized cognitive behavior therapy for obesity (CBT-OB). Currently, the main focus of his research is evaluating CBT-E and CBT-OB in the treatment of adult and adolescent patients with eating disorders and obesity respectively, both in outpatient and in inpatient settings. He is the director of the master course for health professionals '1° Certificate in Eating Disorder and Obesity'. He also teaches CBT-E and CBT-OB at several Italian psychotherapy schools and supervises teams in Europe, the US, Australia, and Middles West. He is the author of several books, book chapters, and about 150 peer review articles; and he is a member of the editorial board of several scientific journals.

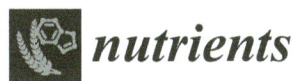

Editorial

Nutrition and Fitness: Mental Health

Riccardo Dalle Grave

Department of Eating and Weight Disorders, Villa Garda Hospital, Via Monte Baldo, 8937016 Garda (VR), Italy;
rdalleg@gmail.com

Received: 15 June 2020; Accepted: 16 June 2020; Published: 17 June 2020

Mental disorders are one of the leading causes of disability, being associated with about 18.9% of years lived with a disability [1]. Traditionally, depressive disorders, bipolar disorders, schizophrenia, anxiety disorders, and eating disorders have been treated with psychopharmacological drugs, including antipsychotics, antidepressants, mood stabilizers, and antianxiety agents, and/or different forms of psychotherapies. Unfortunately, with these treatments, the burden of mental disorders is prevented in less than 50% of cases, an outcome indicating the need to find new additional strategies and procedures to improve their management [2].

Mens sana in corpore sano (a healthy mind in a healthy body) is a Latin phrase taken from Giovenale (Satire, X, 356) that remains relevant and is supported by today's data regarding nutrition and physical activity, and their contribution to mental health. Indeed, several data have found an association between nutrition physical fitness and mental health [2–5], supporting the potential role of using nutrients and physical activity as agents for prevention, treatment, or augmentation of treatment for mental disorders in children, adolescents, and adults.

The Special Issue "Nutrition and Fitness: Mental Health" of *Nutrients* includes four original articles [6–9] and three systematic reviews [10–12]. The first original article assessed the interconnections between specific quality of life domains (assessed with Short Form-36 [SF-36]) in 716 consecutive female and male patients with obesity and high or low physical performance using an innovative statistical analysis based on network approach [6]. Low-performing patients (64.7% of the sample) reported lower quality of life domain scores, but the network structures were similar in the two groups, with the SF-36 Vitality representing the central domain in both networks. Moreover, in patients with obesity and low physical performance levels, mental health was a central variable, indicating that psychological aspects should be considered in defining the quality of life in patients with low physical performance levels.

In the second original article, 162 individuals who were obese or overweight were randomly allocated to four interventions, 24 weeks in duration [8]: strength, endurance, combined strength + endurance, and guideline-based physical activity; all in combination with a 25–30% caloric restriction diet. The study found several positive effects of the intervention on energy intake, macronutrient selection, and body composition changes, with a significant reduction of body mass index and body fat percentage, but no significant differences of exercise type. The study also confirmed that individuals allocated to a long-term exercise program associated with dietary advice do not increase their energy intake in a compensatory fashion.

The third original article randomly allocated 51 patients with multiple sclerosis to 800 mg of epigallocatechin gallate (EGCG) and 60 mL of coconut oil or placebo for four months [7]. Both groups followed the same isocaloric Mediterranean diet. EGCG and coconut oil decreased state anxiety and functional capacity, while the levels of interleukin 6 (IL-6) decreased in both groups, likely because of the antioxidant effect of the Mediterranean diet.

The fourth original article investigated the public health topic of the association between food insecurity (i.e., the presence of limited or uncertain availability or access to nutritionally sufficient, socially relevant, and safe foods) and depressive symptoms in 8613 adults who participated in the

Indonesia Family Life Survey (IFLS) in 2007 and 2014 [9]. The study found a positive association between depressive symptoms and food insecurity: a finding that underlines the importance to implement specific nutritional and health programs to prevent and treat both food insecurity and mental health.

The first systematic reviews synthesized data from 14 studies to assess and discuss the potential role of microbiota-orientated treatments (including fecal microbiota transplantation (FMT) in major depression and schizophrenia) [10]. The results indicate that probiotics seem to have a medium-to-large significant effect on depressive symptoms, but it is not clear if these positive effects are maintained after probiotic discontinuation. Since FTM has been shown to improve microbiota in several gut disorders, the authors suggest that this procedure may be a potential strategy to test for improving the efficacy of microbiota-orientated treatments in major depression and schizophrenia and maintain their effect over time.

In the second systematic review, the authors synthesized the data of 25 studies (ten experimental and 15 observational studies) assessing the relationship between energy balance-related behavior (i.e., physical activity, sedentary, and dietary behavior) and burn-out risk [11]. Physical activity seems effective in reducing burn-out, as supported by the data of nine experimental and 14 studies. On the contrary, although the data of few observational studies suggest that being sedentary and eating less healthily are both associated with higher burn-out risk, there is a need for more high-quality research to reach meaningful conclusions on this association.

However, when the physical activity becomes excessive and compulsive, a distinctive behavioral feature of a subgroup of patients with eating disorders [13], it is associated with more severe general and eating disorder psychopathology, as synthesized by the third systematic review [12] of this Special Issue. The authors, who analyzed 47 articles, suggest using the term "problematic use of physical activity (PPA)" to define this unhealthy form of exercising and propose an original model for the development of PPA in patients with anorexia nervosa, encompassing five periods evolving into three clinical stages. They also suggest the presence of two components of PPA in anorexia nervosa: (i) voluntary PPA to influence body shape and weight; and (ii) involuntary PPA that it is biology driven and increases with weight-loss. Future research will have to test the theory proposed by the Authors and its clinical utility.

In conclusion, the findings of the original articles and systematic reviews of this Special Issue confirm that nutrition and physical activity seem to play an important role in maintaining good mental health and are two potential interventions to improve the management of mental disorders.

Conflicts of Interest: The authors declare no conflict of interest.

References

1. Whiteford, H.A.; Ferrari, A.J.; Degenhardt, L.; Feigin, V.; Vos, T. The global burden of mental, neurological and substance use disorders: An analysis from the Global Burden of Disease Study 2010. *PLoS ONE* **2015**, *10*, e0116820. [CrossRef] [PubMed]
2. Marx, W.; Moseley, G.; Berk, M.; Jacka, F. Nutritional psychiatry: The present state of the evidence. *Proc. Nutr. Soc.* **2017**, *76*, 427–436. [CrossRef] [PubMed]
3. Biddle, S.J.; Asare, M. Physical activity and mental health in children and adolescents: A review of reviews. *Br. J. Sports Med.* **2011**, *45*, 886–895. [CrossRef] [PubMed]
4. Mikkelsen, K.; Stojanovska, L.; Polenakovic, M.; Bosevski, M.; Apostolopoulos, V. Exercise and mental health. *Maturitas* **2017**, *106*, 48–56. [CrossRef] [PubMed]
5. O'Neil, A.; Quirk, S.E.; Housden, S.; Brennan, S.L.; Williams, L.J.; Pasco, J.A.; Berk, M.; Jacka, F.N. Relationship between diet and mental health in children and adolescents: A systematic review. *Am. J. Public Health* **2014**, *104*, e31–e42. [CrossRef] [PubMed]
6. Dalle Grave, R.; Soave, F.; Ruocco, A.; Dametti, L.; Calugi, S. Quality of Life and Physical Performance in Patients with Obesity: A Network Analysis. *Nutrients* **2020**, *12*, 602. [CrossRef] [PubMed]

7. Platero, J.L.; Cuerda-Ballester, M.; Ibáñez, V.; Sancho, D.; Lopez-Rodríguez, M.M.; Drehmer, E.; Ortí, J.E.R. The Impact of Coconut Oil and Epigallocatechin Gallate on the Levels of IL-6, Anxiety and Disability in Multiple Sclerosis Patients. *Nutrients* **2020**, *12*, 305. [CrossRef] [PubMed]
8. Castro, E.A.; Carraça, E.V.; Cupeiro, R.; López-Plaza, B.; Teixeira, P.J.; González-Lamuño, D.; Peinado, A.B. The Effects of the Type of Exercise and Physical Activity on Eating Behavior and Body Composition in Overweight and Obese Subjects. *Nutrients* **2020**, *12*, 557. [CrossRef] [PubMed]
9. Isaura, E.R.; Chen, Y.C.; Adi, A.C.; Fan, H.Y.; Li, C.Y.; Yang, S.H. Association between Depressive Symptoms and Food Insecurity among Indonesian Adults: Results from the 2007-2014 Indonesia Family Life Survey. *Nutrients* **2019**, *11*, 3026. [CrossRef] [PubMed]
10. Fond, G.B.; Lagier, J.C.; Honore, S.; Lancon, C.; Korchia, T.; Sunhary De Verville, P.L.; Llorca, P.M.; Auquier, P.; Guedj, E.; Boyer, L. Microbiota-Orientated Treatments for Major Depression and Schizophrenia. *Nutrients* **2020**, *12*, 1024. [CrossRef] [PubMed]
11. Verhavert, Y.; De Martelaer, K.; Van Hoof, E.; Van Der Linden, E.; Zinzen, E.; Deliens, T. The Association between Energy Balance-Related Behavior and Burn-Out in Adults: A Systematic Review. *Nutrients* **2020**, *12*, 397. [CrossRef] [PubMed]
12. Rizk, M.; Mattar, L.; Kern, L.; Berthoz, S.; Duclos, J.; Viltart, O.; Godart, N. Physical Activity in Eating Disorders: A Systematic Review. *Nutrients* **2020**, *12*, 183. [CrossRef]
13. Dalle Grave, R. Features and management of compulsive exercising in eating disorders. *Phys Sportsmed.* **2009**, *37*, 20–28. [CrossRef] [PubMed]

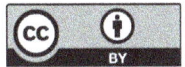

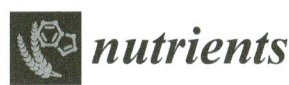

Article

Quality of Life and Physical Performance in Patients with Obesity: A Network Analysis

Riccardo Dalle Grave *, Fabio Soave, Antonella Ruocco, Laura Dametti and Simona Calugi

Department of Eating and Weight Disorders, Villa Garda Hospital, 37138 Garda (VR), Italy;
info@attiviperstarbene.it (F.S.); anto82ruocco@gmail.com (A.R.); lauradametti96@gmail.com (L.D.);
si.calugi@gmail.com (S.C.)
* Correspondence: rdalleg@tin.it

Received: 6 February 2020; Accepted: 24 February 2020; Published: 26 February 2020

Abstract: Background: The aim of this study was to investigate the interconnections between specific quality-of-life domains in patients with obesity and high or low physical performance using a network approach. Methods: 716 consecutive female and male patients (aged 18–65 years) with obesity seeking weight-loss treatment were included. The 36-item Short Form Health Survey (SF-36) and the six-minute walking test (6MWT) were used to assess quality of life and physical performance, respectively. The sample was split into two groups according to the distance walked in the 6MWT. Network structures of the SF-36 domains in the two groups were assessed and compared, and the relative importance of individual items in the network structures was determined using centrality analyses. Results: 35.3% (n = 253) of participants covered more distance than expected, and 64.7% (n = 463) did not. Although low-performing patients showed lower quality of life domain scores, the network structures were similar in the two groups, with the SF-36 Vitality representing the central domain in both networks. Mental Health was a node with strong connections in patients who walked less distance. Conclusions: These findings indicate that psychosocial variables represent the most influential and interconnected features as regards quality of life in both groups.

Keywords: obesity; physical performance; network analysis; vitality; mental health

1. Introduction

Obesity is a condition characterized by an excessive accumulation of fat in adipose tissue; it is linked to an increased risk of chronic diseases, disability, and mortality [1], and is also often associated with poor physical fitness levels, e.g., muscle strength [2], and cardiorespiratory fitness [3]. Moreover, both obesity and physical performance are associated with quality of life. Indeed, a recent systematic review found that in all populations examined, obesity was associated with a significantly worse generic and obesity-specific quality of life [3]. Furthermore, significant weight loss after a bariatric surgery or non-bariatric interventions has been associated with improvements in quality of life [4]. Some evidence also supports a link between quality of life and physical fitness in adolescent patients with obesity, and a recent study indicated cardiorespiratory fitness as the main mediator in the relationship between body mass index (BMI) and quality of life [5]. However, this relationship requires a more in-depth investigation in adults.

Understanding whether specific aspects of quality of life are more prominent or strongly interlinked in patients with obesity with different levels of physical performance is relevant to the design of targeted interventions to promote optimum weight management, and may require innovative methods of investigation, such as network analysis—a novel way of representing variables as complex dynamic systems of interacting variables. The inspection of networks elucidates the extent to which items belonging to the same construct are connected to each other, and the strength of their reciprocal relationships. Although in the majority of applications network analysis typically used to be limited to determining a network structure in a single population, recently the focus has shifted from single-population studies to the research comparing network structures from different subpopulations [6]. To this end, specific tests have been developed [7] to examine whether the network structure is identical across subpopulations, whether specific correlations differ in strength between subpopulations, and whether the overall connectivity is equal across subgroups.

Network analysis had never before been used to examine the empirical relationships between quality of life domains in patients with obesity, and the aim of the present study was therefore to use a network approach to provide benchmark data on the interconnections between specific health and psychological features of the quality of life in patients with high or low levels of physical performance seeking treatment for obesity.

2. Materials and Methods

Participants were recruited from consecutive referrals by family doctors to the rehabilitative treatment programs for obesity at the inpatient unit of the Villa Garda Hospital Department of Eating and Weight Disorders during the years 2016–2019. Patients were eligible for this study if they were aged between 18 and 65 years, had a BMI $\geq$ 30.0 kg/m^2, and at least one weight loss-responsive comorbidity (i.e., type 2 diabetes, cardiovascular disease, sleep apnea, severe joint disease, two or more cardiovascular risk factors), as defined by Adult Treatment Panel III [8]. The criteria for exclusion were pregnancy or lactation, medications that affect body weight, medical comorbidities associated with weight loss, severe psychiatric disorders (i.e., bulimia nervosa, acute psychotic disorders, substance use disorders), use of a walker, and the need in assistance/support with walking.

As per the Italian National Health System's National ethical guidelines, this study was classed as a routine service assessment rather than research per se, as all the procedures used for treatment and assessment were performed as routine clinical practice, and therefore no ethical clearance was necessary. That being said, each patient provided written informed consent to the collection and processing of their anonymous clinical data in the service-level research setting.

All data were collected on the second day of admission to the programs. Specifically, BMI was determined using the standard formula of body weight (kg) divided by height (m^2) following measurement of body weight and height using medical weighing scales (Seca Digital Wheelchair Scale Model 664, Hamburg, Germany) and a stadiometer (Wall-Mounted Mechanical Height Rod Model 00051A; Wunder, REA (MI), Italy), respectively. The scale was calibrated for accuracy by an external accredited laboratory every two months. For the purposes of these measurements, participants were weighed in the morning (12 h after eating) wearing only lightweight clothes and no shoes and standing with minimal movement with hands by their sides. Body weight was measured once for each participant to the nearest 0.1 kg.

Physical performance was assessed by means of the six-minute walking test (6MWT) [9] according to international guidelines [10]. The 6MWT was performed along a 20 m long corridor in the department, marked with tape on the floor every 2 m; starting and finishing points were also marked on the floor in a similar fashion. Before the start and at the end of each test, pulse, respiratory rate, and oxygen saturation were measured. The patients were instructed to walk as fast as they could, but were allowed to stop or rest during the test if necessary. All participants concluded the test without breaks. The specific reference equation for predicting distance walked in six minutes in adult subjects with obesity [9] was used to assess the difference between the predicted and real 6MWT scores. The patients walking as far as or farther than predicted were included in Group H (i.e., obesity with a higher 6MWT score than expected), and the patients walking less than predicted were allocated to Group L (i.e., obesity with a lower 6MWT score than expected).

The quality of life was assessed using the validated Italian version of the Short Form-36 (SF-36)—a generic health related quality-of-life questionnaire [11,12]. The SF-36 incorporates questions about (role) functioning and satisfaction with various life domains; it consists of 36 questions, and assesses four domains related to the physical component of quality of life (Physical Functioning, Physical

Role Functioning, Bodily Pain, General Health Perception), and four domains related to the mental component (Vitality, Social Functioning, Emotional Role Functioning, and Mental Health). SF-36 scale scores range from 0 to 100; a higher score indicates a better quality of life.

Statistical Analysis

Variables are presented as means and standard deviations, or frequencies and percentages, as appropriate. Either the *t*-test or the chi-squared test was used to compare Group L and Group H, as appropriate. Network analysis was performed on the 8 SF-36 domain scores for each group, thereby creating a graphical representation of the interconnections between SF-36 domains; domains are depicted as nodes, while their intercorrelations are represented as lines, or "edges"—the thicker and more saturated the edge, the stronger the correlation. The network display is based on an algorithm [13] that places strongly associated nodes at the center of the network and weakly associated nodes at the periphery. To reduce the number of false-positive edges, the Least Absolute Shrinkage and Selection Operator (LASSO) was applied. It estimates small or unstable correlations as zero, and thereby creates a conservative model; this way, the network edges that are less likely to be genuine are removed, and the network is easier to interpret.

Once a collection of networks had been obtained, we minimized the Extended Bayesian Information Criterion (EBIC) [14] to optimize their fit; this process is a particularly effective means of revealing the true network structure [15,16], especially when the generating network is sparse (i.e., does not contain many edges).

To quantify the importance of each node in the network, we then calculated the betweenness, closeness, and strength centrality indices. The betweenness denotes the number of times a specific node acts as a bridge along the shortest path between two nodes, while the closeness measures the number of direct and indirect links between each node and the others; the strength of these inter-node connections is expressed as the degree. [17]. Each of these indices were normalized (mean = 0, and standard deviation (SD) = 1), so that an index value of > 1 indicates that it is > 1 SD from the mean.

Data management and descriptive analyses were performed using SPSS version 26, and the network analysis—using the JASP version 0.10.2 statistical software (Department of Psychological Methods University of Amsterdam, Amsterdam, The Netherlands, https://jasp-stats.org/).The R-package NetworkComparisonTest was used to test the invariant network structure, the invariant edge strength, and the invariant global strength between subgroups [7].

3. Results

3.1. Patient characteristics

Of the 716 patients recruited, 35.3% (*n* = 253) covered more distance in the 6MWT than predicted, and 64.7% (*n* = 463) did not. On the basis of these distances, the patients were allocated to Groups H and L, respectively. The two groups had similar age, BMI and waist circumference. However, Group H patients had greater body weight and higher scores in all SF-36 domains than those in Group L. A greater proportion of males than females reached a higher 6MWT score than expected (Table 1).

Table 1. Demographic and clinical characteristics of patients with obesity walking as far as or farther than predicted during the six-minute walking test (Group H), and of patients with obesity walking less than predicted during the six-minute walking test (Group L). Data are presented as mean ± SD or number (%), as appropriate.

	Group L (*n* = 463)	Group H (*n* = 253)	*t*-Test or Chi-Squared Test	*p*-Value
Gender				
Female	357 (77.1%)	101 (22.1%)	98.1	<0.001
Male	106 (22.9%)	152 (77.9%)		
Age, years	51.1 ± 12.3	50.1 ± 10.5	1.17	0.244
Body weight, kg	112.7 ± 24.8	123.0 ± 24.4	5.36	<0.001
Body mass index, kg/m^2	41.8 ± 8.0	41.5 ± 6.8	0.46	0.644
Waist circumference, cm	124.2 ±19.3	126.5 ± 18.3	1.51	0.132
Short Form-36				
Physical Functioning	54.9 ± 26.2	71.8 ± 20.8	9.39	<0.001
Physical Role Functioning	51.1 ± 40.7	65.7 ± 38.1	4.64	<0.001
Bodily Pain	50.3 ± 27.4	65.5 ± 25.3	7.31	<0.001
General Health Perception	46.9 ± 19.1	55.7 ± 20.4	5.35	<0.001
Vitality	46.9 ± 20.6	54.1 ± 18.0	4.62	<0.001
Social Functioning	62.4 ± 26.2	67.4 ± 24.4	2.47	0.014
Emotional Role Functioning	60.6 ± 42.3	70.3 ± 39.0	2.97	0.003
Mental Health	60.0 ± 20.6	65.9 ± 17.7	4.04	<0.001

3.2. Network structure in Group L and Group H

The network analysis was carried out on the overall sample, which included 253 Group H patients and 463 Group L patients. The network structure confirmed that SF-36 physical and mental components, colored in black and white, respectively, comprised two distinct clusters in both Groups (Figure 1). Groups H and L displayed similar values for the maximum difference in all of the edge weights of the networks (M = 0.30, *p* = 0.11). Moreover, the difference in global strength between the networks was not significant (S = 0.18, *p* = 0.82).

Concerning the centrality of SF-36 domains, two domains played a key role. In Group H, Physical Functioning and Vitality had the highest betweenness (directly connecting more items with each other) and closeness (direct and indirect connections with other items), and Vitality had the highest degree (stronger links with other items). On the other hand, in Group L, Emotional Role Functioning and Physical Role Functioning had the highest betweenness, whereas Vitality had highest closeness, and Vitality and Mental Health the highest degrees (stronger links with other items).

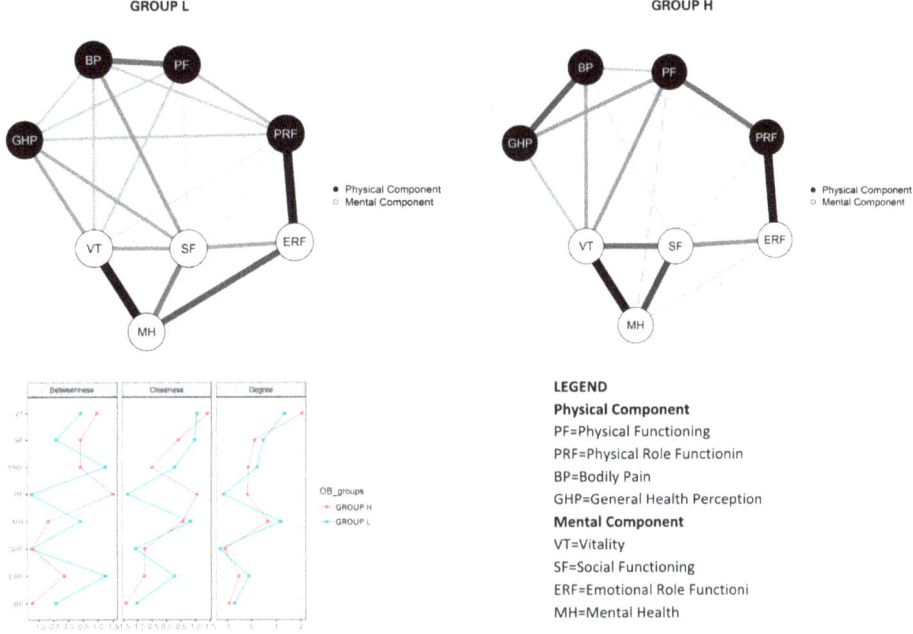

Figure 1. The network of SF-36 quality-of-life domains for patients with obesity walking less than predicted during the six-minute walking test (Group L, on the left), and for patients with obesity walking as far as or farther than predicted during the six-minute walking test (Group H, on the right), and their respective centrality indices (panel C: red line = Group L; blue line = Group H).

4. Discussion

This study aimed to evaluate the interconnections between quality-of-life domains in patients with obesity and either low or high physical performance levels using a network approach. This innovative analysis revealed three main findings. Firstly, about two-thirds of patients with obesity walked a smaller distance than expected. This could be attributed to the severity of clinical features in our sample, which was comprised of patients seeking treatment for obesity in an inpatient setting, and could indicate that their reduced functional capacity was due to comorbid conditions associated with obesity [9].

The second finding concerns the differences between the two groups. As expected, the lower-performing patients had a lower quality of life than those who walked farther than predicted, confirming that physical functioning and quality of life are associated in both the physical and mental domains of the latter.

Our third finding indicated that the network structures of low- and high-performing patients seeking treatment for obesity are invariant. This indicates that the key elements for evaluating the quality of life in a person with obesity are similar, regardless of their physical performance level. In both networks, Vitality (a domain including items investigating pep/life, energy, worn out, tired) plays a key role and represents the domain with the strongest connections with all the other domains, indicating the importance of this variable in the perception of quality of life. In low-performing patients, Mental Health (a domain including items investigating nervous, down in dumps, peaceful, blue/sad, happy) was found to be a key variable, too, suggesting that patients with low physical performance tend to judge their quality of life based mainly on psychological variables, and seem less interested in physical variables. This could, in part, explain the less attention to maintaining good physical performance in this subgroup of patients with obesity.

The study has two main strengths. Firstly, to our knowledge, it is the first to apply network analysis to investigate the relationships between quality of life domains in patients with obesity, and to explore the network structure and strength of relationships between quality of life domains as related to lower and higher physical performance levels. Secondly, the fact that we used the 6MWT to measure performance means that the study would be easy to replicate. Testing the ability to walk a distance is a quick and inexpensive measure of physical function, and an important component of quality of life, since it reflects the capacity to undertake day-to-day activities.

However, the study also has certain weaknesses. Firstly, it was a cross-sectional study measuring quality of life during a single examination session, and we cannot therefore draw conclusions about the association between physical performance and quality of life in the management of obesity over time. Secondly, while we have routinely measured pulse, oxygen, and respiratory rates during the 6MWT, we have not collected these data in the data set, and therefore we do not have accurate information about these variables of physical fitness. Thirdly, generalizing these study's findings beyond this inpatient population should be attempted with caution, because our sample may not be representative of patients with obesity seeking treatment in other settings, such as outpatient treatment, or subjects with obesity not seeking treatment.

5. Conclusions

Network comparisons provided interesting insight into the most interlinked quality of life domains in patients with obesity and low and high physical performance levels, revealing similar network structures, with Vitality playing a central role among quality of life variables. Moreover, in patients with obesity and low physical performance levels, Mental Health is a central variable, indicating that psychological aspects should be considered in defining quality of life in patients with low physical performance levels. Knowledge of these aspects can provide a useful guide for clinicians, suggesting the use of psychosocial interventions and improving the importance of physical fitness aspects in obesity management, especially in patients with low physical performance. Future studies should contribute to clarifying the relationship between quality of life and physical performance using new statistical approaches, including network analysis. Moreover, well-conducted longitudinal clinical trials and intervention studies should be performed to evaluate the effect of associating strategies to improve mental health on the standard weight management in improving physical fitness and quality of life of patients with obesity.

Author Contributions: Conceptualization, R.D.G. and S.C.; data curation, S.C., F.S., A.R., L.D.; formal analysis, S.C.; investigation, R.D.G.; methodology, R.D.G. and S.C.; resources, R.D.G., S.C., F.S., A.R., L.D.; software, S.C.; writing—review and editing, R.D.G., S.C., F.S., A.R., L.D. All authors have read and agreed to the published version of the manuscript.

Funding: This research received no external funding.

Conflicts of Interest: The authors declare that they are aware of no conflict of interest.

References

1. Afshin, A.; Forouzanfar, M.H.; Reitsma, M.B.; Sur, P.; Estep, K.; Lee, A.; Marczak, L.; Mokdad, A.H.; Moradi-Lakeh, M.; Naghavi, M.; et al. Health Effects of Overweight and Obesity in 195 Countries over 25 Years. *N. Engl. J. Med.* **2017**, *377*, 13–27. [CrossRef] [PubMed]
2. El Ghoch, M.; Rossi, A.P.; Calugi, S.; Rubele, S.; Soave, F.; Zamboni, M.; Chignola, E.; Mazzali, G.; Bazzani, P.V.; Dalle Grave, R. Physical performance measures in screening for reduced lean body mass in adult females with obesity. *Nutr. Metab. Cardiovasc. Dis. NMCD* **2018**, *28*, 917–921. [CrossRef] [PubMed]
3. Kokkinos, P.; Faselis, C.; Franklin, B.; Lavie, C.J.; Sidossis, L.; Moore, H.; Karasik, P.; Myers, J. Cardiorespiratory fitness, body mass index and heart failure incidence. *Eur. J. Heart Fail.* **2019**, *21*, 436–444. [CrossRef] [PubMed]

4. Kroes, M.; Osei-Assibey, G.; Baker-Searle, R.; Huang, J. Impact of weight change on quality of life in adults with overweight/obesity in the United States: A systematic review. *Curr. Med. Res. Opin.* **2016**, *32*, 485–508. [CrossRef] [PubMed]

5. Evaristo, S.; Moreira, C.; Santos, R.; Lopes, L.; Abreu, S.; Agostinis-Sobrinho, C.; Oliveira-Santos, J.; Mota, J. Associations between health-related quality of life and body mass index in Portuguese adolescents: LabMed physical activity study. *Int. J. Adolesc. Med. Health* **2018**, *31*. [CrossRef] [PubMed]

6. van Borkulo, C.; Boschloo, L.; Borsboom, D.; Penninx, B.W.; Waldorp, L.J.; Schoevers, R.A. Association of Symptom Network Structure With the Course of [corrected] Depression. *JAMA Psychiatry* **2015**, *72*, 1219–1226. [CrossRef] [PubMed]

7. Van Borkulo, C.; Boschloo, L.; Kossakowski, J.; Tio, P.; Schoevers, R.; Borsboom, D.; Waldorp, L.J. Comparing Network Structures on Three Aspects: A Permutation Test. Available online: https://www.researchgate.net/publication/314750838_Comparing_network_structures_on_three_aspects_A_permutation_test (accessed on 28 January 2020).

8. Expert Panel on Detection; Evaluation; Treatment of High Blood Cholesterol in Adults. Executive Summary of the Third Report of the National Cholesterol Education Program (NCEP) Expert Panel on Detection, Evaluation, and Treatment of High Blood Cholesterol In Adults (Adult Treatment Panel III). *JAMA* **2001**, *285*, 2486–2497. [CrossRef] [PubMed]

9. Capodaglio, P.; De Souza, S.A.; Parisio, C.; Precilios, H.; Vismara, L.; Cimolin, V.; Brunani, A. Reference values for the 6-Min Walking Test in obese subjects. *Disabil. Rehabil.* **2013**, *35*, 1199–1203. [CrossRef] [PubMed]

10. ATS statement: Guidelines for the six-minute walk test. *Am. J. Respir. Crit. Care Med.* **2002**, *166*, 111–117. [CrossRef] [PubMed]

11. McHorney, C.A.; Ware, J.E., Jr.; Raczek, A.E. The MOS 36-Item Short-Form Health Survey (SF-36): II. Psychometric and clinical tests of validity in measuring physical and mental health constructs. *Med. Care* **1993**, *31*, 247–263. [CrossRef] [PubMed]

12. Apolone, G.; Mosconi, P. The Italian SF-36 Health Survey: Translation, validation and norming. *J. Clin. Epidemiol.* **1998**, *51*, 1025–1036. [CrossRef]

13. Fruchterman, T.M.J.; Reingold, E.M. Graph drawing by force-directed placement. *Softw. Pract. Exp.* **1991**, *21*, 1129–1164. [CrossRef]

14. Chen, J.; Chen, Z. Extended Bayesian information criteria for model selection with large model spaces. *Biometrika* **2008**, *95*, 759–771. [CrossRef]

15. Foygel, R.; Drton, M. Extended Bayesian Information Criteria for Gaussian Graphical Models. In *Advances in Neural Information Processing Systems 23*; Lafferty, J.D., Williams, C.K.I., Shawe-Taylor, J., Zemel, R.S., Culotta, A., Eds.; Curran Associates, Inc.: Reed Hook, NY, USA, 2010; pp. 604–612.

16. Barber, R.F.; Drton, M. High-dimensional Ising model selection with Bayesian information criteria. *Electron. J. Stat.* **2015**, *9*, 567–607. [CrossRef]

17. Borsboom, D.; Cramer, A.O. Network analysis: An integrative approach to the structure of psychopathology. *Annu. Rev. Clin. Psychol.* **2013**, *9*, 91–121. [CrossRef] [PubMed]

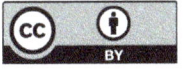

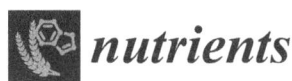

Article

The Effects of the Type of Exercise and Physical Activity on Eating Behavior and Body Composition in Overweight and Obese Subjects

Eliane A. Castro [1,2], Eliana V. Carraça [3], Rocío Cupeiro [2], Bricia López-Plaza [4], Pedro J. Teixeira [3], Domingo González-Lamuño [5,*] and Ana B. Peinado [2] on behalf of the PRONAF Study Group

[1] Department of Sports Sciences and Physical Conditioning, Faculty of Education, Universidad Católica de la Santísima Concepción, Concepción 4090541, Chile; elianeaparecidacastro@gmail.com
[2] LFE Research Group, Faculty of Physical Activity and Sport Sciences, Universidad Politécnica de Madrid, 28040 Madrid, Spain; rocio.cupeiro@upm.es (R.C.); anabelen.peinado@upm.es (A.B.P.)
[3] Interdisciplinary Centre for the Study of Human Performance (CIPER), Faculdade de Motricidade Humana, Universidade de Lisboa, 1495-688 Lisbon, Portugal; elianacarraca@gmail.com (E.V.C.); pteixeira@fmh.ulisboa.pt (P.J.T.)
[4] Nutrition Department, Hospital La Paz Institute for Health Research (IdiPAZ), 28046 Madrid, Spain; bricia.plaza@idipaz.es
[5] Department of Pediatrics, University of Cantabria-University Hospital Marqués de Valdecilla, 39008 Santander, Spain
* Correspondence: gonzaleld@unican.es; Tel.: +34-942-202604

Received: 1 January 2020; Accepted: 17 February 2020; Published: 20 February 2020

Abstract: The aim of this study was to examine whether a type of exercise favors better compliance with a prescribed diet, higher eating-related motivation, healthier diet composition or greater changes in body composition in overweight and obese subjects. One hundred and sixty-two (males $n = 79$), aged 18–50 years, were randomized into four intervention groups during 24 weeks: strength, endurance, combined strength + endurance and guideline-based physical activity; all in combination with a 25–30% caloric restriction diet. A food frequency questionnaire and a "3-day food and drink record" were applied pre- and post-intervention. Diet and exercise-related motivation levels were evaluated with a questionnaire developed for this study. Body composition was assessed by DXA and habitual physical activity was measured by accelerometry. Body weight, body mass index (BMI) and body fat percentage decreased and lean body mass increased after the intervention, without differences by groups. No interactions were observed between intervention groups and time; all showing a decreased in energy intake ($p < 0.001$). Carbohydrate and protein intakes increased, and fat intake decreased from pre- to post-intervention without significant interactions with intervention groups, BMI category or gender ($p < 0.001$). Diet-related motivation showed a tendency to increase from pre- to post-intervention (70.0 ± 0.5 vs 71.0 ± 0.6, $p = 0.053$), without significant interactions with intervention groups, BMI or gender. Regarding motivation for exercise, gender x time interactions were observed ($F_{(1,146)} = 7.452$, $p = 0.007$): Women increased their motivation after the intervention (pre: 17.6 ± 0.3, post: 18.2 ± 0.3), while men maintained it. These findings suggest that there are no substantial effects of exercise type on energy intake, macronutrient selection or body composition changes. After a six-month weight loss program, individuals did not reduce their motivation related to diet or exercise, especially women. Individuals who initiate a long-term exercise program do not increase their energy intake in a compensatory fashion, if diet advices are included.

Keywords: macronutrients; energy intake; motivation to diet; motivation to exercise; weight loss program

---

1. Introduction

Obesity is a public health problem, given it relates numerous risk factors for cardiovascular disease and comorbidities [1]; this points out the need for further studies. It is known that healthy habits of physical activity and nutrition work together to maintain body weight at desirable levels [2]. Although diet contributes to a greater extent for short-term weight loss [3], exercise seems to be important in maintaining this loss [4]. Thus, exercise might also facilitate long-term adherence to healthy eating habits and behaviors.

Several studies have analyzed if exercise was able to modulate food intake [5,6], indicating that participation in physical activity as well as its duration and intensity, could contribute to appetite regulation [7], total calorie intake [8] and macronutrient composition of the diet [9,10], resulting in an appropriate energy balance. Other studies have also shown an association between regular physical activity and psychosocial and motivational factors related to a healthier eating behavior [11,12].

However, the type of exercise that can induce greater physiological and behavioral changes, related to eating behavior and food intake, remains unclear. It appears that long-term exercise interventions (more than 1 month) could decrease daily energy intake [5]. Regarding the intensity of effort, some authors found that more intense exercise reduced feelings of hunger during and after its practice [10]. Other authors have shown that absolute caloric intake was superior in high-intensity exercise, compared to moderate-intensity exercise [8]. In terms of the mode of exercise, most studies involved aerobic exercises and regular weight individuals [8,10], and the results are not very consistent. In addition, the literature lacks studies on the relationship between exercise and long-term diet adherence, and that consider the composition of the diet. Therefore, the present study aimed at examining if there is a type of exercise or a physical activity threshold (daily steps' categories) that favors a better compliance with the prescribed diet, a higher eating-related motivation, and a healthier diet composition in overweight and obese subjects.

2. Methods

2.1. Participants

Data for this study were derived from the Nutrition and Physical Activity for Obesity Treatment (PRONAF). The inclusion criteria specified adult subjects, aged 18 to 50 years, who were overweight or obese ($25 \text{ kg/m}^2 \leq$ body mass index [BMI] $\leq 34.9 \text{ kg/m}^2$), sedentary (<30 min physical activity/day and no participation in systematic strength or endurance training—moderate to high intensity more than once a week—in the year prior to the start of the study), normoglycemic, non-smoking and, if females, with regular menstrual cycles. Furthermore, participants with orthopedic limitations, records of stroke, eating disorders such as anorexia, bulimia etc., or any other diseases or medications that could have an effect on performance were also excluded from the study. From the 180 participants that comply with at least 90% of the training sessions and an 80% adherence to the diet total, 162 subjects were included in the analyses regarding the influence of type of exercise and 91 participants in the analyses concerning the influence of physical activity. All participants signed a written informed consent. The PRONAF study was approved by the Human Research Review Committee of the University Hospital La Paz (HULP) (No.NCT01116856).

2.2. Study Design and Intervention

The intervention lasted 22 weeks and the assessments took place one week before (baseline) and after (post) the intervention. Subjects were randomized by drawing lots to compose to one of the four intervention groups—strength training (S), endurance training (E), combined strength + endurance training (SE) and a guideline-based physical activity (PA), assuring a homogeneous distribution of age and gender among groups. The complete methodology and the diagram flow can be found in Zapico et al. [13].

2.2.1. Exercise Protocols

The PA group followed general physical activity recommendations from the American College of Sports Medicine [14]. These recommendations were transmitted to the participants via a personal meeting. Exercise from this group was not supervised, like a classical intervention. Subjects in the S, E, and SE groups trained three times per week. All training sessions were carefully supervised by certified personal trainers. The exercise programs were designed according to the subject's muscle strength and heart rate reserve (Figure 1). All exercise programs were performed in circuit. Adherence to exercise was calculated by the number of sessions completed in regard to the theoretical sessions ([sessions performed /total sessions] × 100).

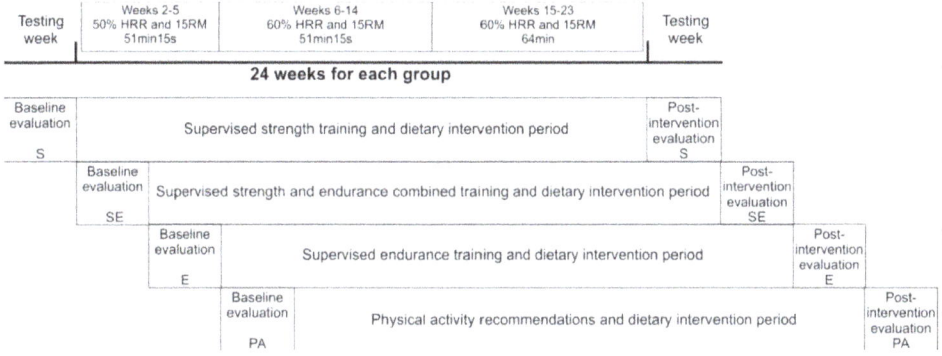

Figure 1. Time line of the Study. HRR: heart rate reserve; RM: repetition maximum; S: strength training group; E: endurance training group; SE: combined strength plus endurance training group; PA: physical activity recommendations group.

2.2.2. Hypocaloric Diet

All participants underwent an individualized dietary intervention based on a hypocaloric diet (25–30% reduction on the total daily energy expenditure) by expert dieticians. Macronutrient distribution was set according to the Spanish Society of Community Nutrition recommendations [15].

2.3. Assessments

2.3.1. Physical Activity

Habitual physical activity was measured using the SenseWear Pro3 ArmbandTM (Body Media, Pittsburgh, PA, USA) and data inclusion followed the criteria published elsewhere [16]. Three daily steps' categories considering initial data (before intervention) were established (<7500, 7500–10,000, >10,000 steps) [17]. The accelerometer recorded PA in metabolic equivalents (METs) for each 60 s time window (60 s epochs). Physical activity level was calculated using the average from the 3 valid days and expressed as MET per day. The daily energy expenditure was calculated using the Body Media propriety algorithm (Innerview Research Software Version 6.0, Body Media, Pittsburgh, PA, USA).

2.3.2. Eating Behavior

All food and beverages consumed by the participants were recorded using a food frequency questionnaire and a "three-day food and drink record" [18]. Also, participants were asked to measure the amount of food consumed with household measurements (e.g., cups, teaspoons, tablespoons) or to write down the quantity written on commercial packaging. The total energy intake (TEI) or kilocalories consumed in the diet and macronutrient percentages (carbohydrate [CHO], fat and protein [PRO]) were calculated using the DIAL software (Alce Ingeniería S.L., Madrid, Spain). Diet compliance was calculated as the estimated Kcal of the diet (provided by dieticians) divided by the real Kcal intake ([estimated kcal of diet/real Kcal intake] 100), representing perfect adherence values equal to 100.

2.3.3. Motivation

Motivation was evaluated with a questionnaire specifically developed for this study. This questionnaire consisted of 10 questions, rated on a 10-point Likert-type scale. Eight questions were related to diet motivation and two remaining to exercise motivation. Participants punctuated their diet-related motivation on a scale of de 0 to 10 by answering the following questions: "What is your motivation … " (1) to make changes in diet; (2) to go to dietary control appointments; (3) to reduce fat consumption (sausages, sauces, breaded, snacks, etc.); (4) to reduce the consumption of sugars (candies, chocolates, cakes, etc.); (5) to reduce the consumption of alcohol (if the participant did not consume alcohol, he should punctuate 10); (6) to increase fruit consumption; (7) to increase consumption of vegetables; (8) to increase fish consumption. Also, subjects scored their exercise-related motivation by answering the following questions: "What is your motivation … " (1) to exercise regularly; (2) to perform the physical exercise tasks recommended in the program. The total scores for diet and exercise-related motivation were calculated by summing the scores of the respective questions. Subscales of motivations to diet and exercise showed acceptable internal consistency, with Cronbach's alphas of 0.73, and 0.84, respectively.

2.3.4. Body Composition

Body composition was assessed by dual-energy X-ray absorptiometry scan (DXA) (GE Lunar Prodigy; GE Healthcare, Madison, WI, USA). Height was measured using a Seca Stadiometer (Quirumed, Valencia, Spain), which has a range of 80–200 cm. Body mass was measured using a TANITA BC-420MA balance (Bio Lógica Tecnología Médica S.L, Barcelona, Spain).

2.4. Statistical Procedures

Data are presented as mean ± SD. One-way analysis of variance (ANOVA) was used to analyze differences at baseline among the four intervention groups. Four-way repeated measures ANOVA were used to determine differences among the four intervention groups or among the three daily steps' categories, BMI categories and gender by time. Bonferroni post-hoc tests were employed to locate specific differences. Partial eta-squared (η_P^2) was adopted for interactions and small, moderate and large effect corresponded to values equal or greater than 0.001, 0.059, and 0.138, respectively [19]. Effect sizes (ES) were calculated by Cohen's d and interpretation based on <0.2 = trivial, ≥0.2<0.5 = small effect, ≥0.5<0.8 = moderate effect, and ≥0.8 = large effect. Pearson's correlations separated by intervention groups were used to test associations between eating behavior, physical activity and motivations changes. All analyses were conducted in SPSS-PC v20 (IBM SPSS Statistics, Armonk, NY USA), and level of significance was set at 0.05.

3. Results

Participants' baseline characteristics are described in Table 1. No differences were observed among intervention groups for any variable.

Large negative correlations between diet compliance and TEI were observed in all intervention groups ($p < 0.001$). Moderate to large correlations between motivations to diet and to exercise were also observed in all groups ($p < 0.05$), except in the strength group (Table 2).

Analysis of variance showed that all intervention groups, similarly, decreased body weight ($F_{(1,143)} = 661.636$, $p < 0.001$, ES = 0.58), BMI ($F_{(1,143)} = 424.586$, $p < 0.001$, ES = 0.96) and body fat percentage ($F_{(1,143)} = 485.434$, $p < 0.001$, ES = 0.79) and increased lean body mass ($F_{(1,143)} = 484.113$, $p < 0.001$, ES = 0.78). Men had greater body weight and lean body mass and smaller body fat percentage than women before and after the intervention ($p < 0.001$). The remaining interactions and factors were not significant (Figure 2).

Moreover, gender-time interactions ($F_{(1,137)} = 4.783$, $p = 0.030$, $\eta_P^2 = 0.034$) and BMI category-time interactions ($F_{(1,137)} = 13.233$, $p < 0.001$, $\eta_P^2 = 0.088$) for TEI were observed. Men consumed more calories in both, pre- and post-intervention than women (differences: 615.6 kcal, $p < 0.001$, ES = 0.72; 314.0 kcal, $p = 0.002$, ES = 0.66; respectively). Obese subjects showed greater TEI than overweight participants in pre- and post-intervention (differences: 685.6 kcal, $p < 0.001$, ES = 0.81; 176.9 kcal, $p = 0.029$, ES = 0.36; respectively). However, no interactions were observed between intervention groups and time and all of them decreased energy intake ($F_{(1,137)} = 133.742$, $p < 0.001$, ES = 1.06). The remaining interactions and factors were not significant. CHO and PRO intakes increased and fat intake decreased from pre- to post-intervention (CHO: $F_{(1,137)} = 65.652$, $p < 0.001$, ES = 0.81; PRO: $F_{(1,137)} = 90.606$, $p < 0.001$, ES = 1.02; fat: $F_{(1,137)} = 116.561$, $p < 0.001$, ES = 1.16) without significant interactions with intervention groups, BMI category or gender (Figure 3). The remaining interactions and factors were not significant. Diet-related motivation showed a tendency to increase from pre to post-intervention ($F_{(1,146)} = 3.799$, $p = 0.053$, ES = 0.14), without significant interactions with intervention groups, BMI category or gender. In relation to motivation to exercise, interactions between gender and time were observed ($F_{(1,146)} = 7.452$, $p = 0.007$, $\eta_P^2 = 0.049$), and only women increased their motivation after the intervention (pre: 17.6 ± 2.5, post: 18.3 ± 2.0, $p = 0.034$, ES = 0.31). There was a tendency of interactions between intervention group and time ($F_{(3,146)} = 2.440$, $p = 0.067$, $\eta_P^2 = 0.048$) and pairwise comparisons showed that only the PA group decreased motivation to exercise ($p = 0.045$, ES = 0.25). No interactions with BMI category were observed. The remaining interactions and factors were not significant (Figure 4).

When the sample was analyzed by daily steps categories ($n = 91$) similar results were observed. Anthropometric and body composition changes were in the same direction as observed for intervention groups, without differences among daily step categories: Body weight, BMI and body fat percentage decreased and lean body mass increased ($p < 0.05$). BMI category-time interactions were also observed for TEI, and obese individuals obtained greater values than overweight in the pre-intervention (difference: 765.4 kcal, $p = 0.004$, ES = 0.78). However, no interactions were observed between daily step categories and time and all of them decreased energy intake ($p < 0.05$). In addition, as observed earlier, CHO and PRO increased and fat decreased ($p < 0.05$). However, individuals who started the intervention program with more daily steps increased PRO compared to individuals who performed less than 7500 daily steps, independently of BMI category or gender ($\geq 7500 < 10000$: $p = 0.011$, ES = 0.69; ≥ 10000: $p < 0.001$, ES = 1.54). The observed tendency towards an increase in diet-related motivation in all intervention groups was, in this case, significant ($p < 0.05$) without interactions with daily steps' categories, BMI category or gender. Gender-time interaction was also found for motivation to exercise and only women increased their motivation after the intervention (pre: 17.8 ± 2.4, post: 18.8 ± 1.8, $p = 0.011$, ES = 0.47). The remaining interactions and factors were not significant (Table 3).

Table 1. Baseline characteristics.

Variables	S (*n* = 39)	E (*n* = 48)	SE (*n* = 42)	PA (*n* = 33)	F (*p*)
Male (%)	46.2	41.7	50.0	60.6	0.399 [§]
Age (yrs)	38.1 ± 8.9	37.4 ± 7.9	38.7 ± 6.6	38.4 ± 7.9	0.223 (0.88)
Body weight (kg)	88.5 ± 12.5	84.3 ± 11.2	88.8 ± 15.6	88.5 ± 12.6	1.264 (0.29)
Height (cm)	169.5 ± 9.8	167.9 ± 9.1	170.2 ± 10.3	169.5 ± 9.4	0.474 (0.70)
Body mass index (kg/m^2)	30.7 ± 2.2	30.4 ± 2.6	30.2 ± 3.1	30.8 ± 2.6	0.399 (0.75)
Body Fat (%)	41.4 ± 6.0	41.2 ± 6.2	40.8 ± 7.0	40.6 ± 5.7	0.158 (0.92)
Lean body mass (%)	56.7 ± 5.7	56.9 ± 5.8	57.3 ± 6.6	57.5 ± 5.4	0.156 (0.93)
Total Energy Intake (kcal)	2578.4 ± 964.0	2598.74 ± 1122.8	2412.2 ± 727.0	2512.3 ± 709.2	0.335 (0.80)
PAL (METs/day)	1.4 ± 0.2	1.3 ± 0.2	1.4 ± 0.2	1.3 ± 0.1	0.785 (0.50)
Number of steps (steps/day)	11231.5 ± 3648.7	10130.1 ± 3760.1	10064.5 ± 3134.2	9409.6 ± 2189.3	1.010 (0.39)

Data are presented as mean ± SD. S: strength training group; E: endurance training group; SE: combined strength plus endurance training group; PA: physical activity recommendations group; PAL: physical activity level; METs: metabolic equivalents. [§] Chi-Square statistics.

Table 2. Pearson's correlations between changes in dietary variables, motivation and physical activity.

	STRENGTH GROUP					AEROBIC GROUP				
	TEI	Diet Compliance	MVPA	Motivation to Diet	Motivation to Exercise	TEI	Diet Compliance	MVPA	Motivation to Diet	Motivation to Exercise
TEI	1					1				
Diet compliance	−0.93 **	1				−0.88 **	1			
MVPA	0.46 *	−0.26	1			−0.15	0.14	1		
Motivation to diet	0.10	−0.18	−0.22	1		−0.03	−0.09	0.33	1	
Motivation to exercise	0.28	−0.33 *	−0.15	0.18	1	0.08	−0.10	0.07	0.49 **	1
	COMBINED GROUP					PHYSICAL ACTIVITY GROUP				
TEI	1					1				
Diet compliance	−0.88 **	1				−0.92 **	1			
MVPA	0.28	−0.14	1			−0.33	0.65 *	1		
Motivation to diet	−0.13	0.10	−0.01	1		0.29	−0.28	−0.10	1	
Motivation to exercise	0.04	−0.07	0.01	0.42 *	1	0.15	−0.08	0.03	0.43 *	1

TEI: total energy intake; MVPA: moderate-to-vigorous physical activity. * $p < 0.05$; ** $p < 0.001$.

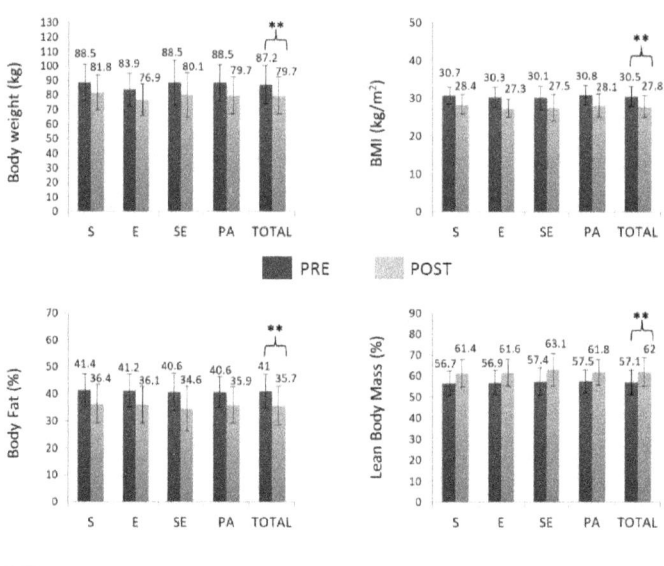

** $p < 0.001$

Figure 2. Anthropometric characteristics and body composition before and after the intervention. BMI: body mass index; S: strength training group; E: endurance training group; SE: combined strength plus endurance training group; PA: physical activity recommendations group.

Table 3. Dietary and motivation-related variables by categories of daily steps at baseline.

	<7500	≥7500<10,000	≥10,000	Total	F	p	η_p^2
Body Weight (kg)							
Baseline	89.1 ± 12.9	84.7 ± 10.6	85.2 ± 13.2	85.8 ± 13.2	T = 419.333	<0.001	0.841
Post-intervention	80.6 ± 11.8	76.6 ± 10.8	77.4 ± 12.9	77.4 ± 12.9 **	TxS = 5.149	0.026	0.061
					TxBMI = 1.008	0.318	0.013
					TxC = 0.176	0.839	0.004
					TxSxBMIxC = 1.444	0.242	0.035
BMI (kg/m^2)							
Baseline	30.5 ± 2.6	29.7 ± 2.2	30.3 ± 2.7	30.1 ± 2.5	T = 313.006	<0.001	0.798
Post-intervention	27.5 ± 2.6	26.7 ± 2	27.3 ± 2.8	27.1 ± 2.5 **	TxS = 0.699	0.406	0.009
					TxBMI = 1.368	0.246	0.017
					TxC = 0.139	0.871	0.003
					TxSxBMIxC = 1.231	0.297	0.030
Body Fat (%)							
Baseline	41.3 ± 5.9	39.2 ± 6.4	40.8 ± 6.6	40.3 ± 6.4	T = 299.511	<0.001	0.791
Post-intervention	35.7 ± 7.1	33.5 ± 7.1	34.6 ± 7.2	34.4 ± 7.1 **	TxS = 2.327	0.131	0.029
					TxBMI = 0.597	0.442	0.007
					TxC = 0.262	0.770	0.007
					TxSxBMIxC = 0.691	0.504	0.017
Lean Body Mass (%)							
Baseline	56.9 ± 5.5	58.8 ± 6.1	57.3 ± 6.2	57.7 ± 6.0	T = 300.088	<0.001	0.792
Post-intervention	62.1 ± 6.6	64.1 ± 6.7	63.1 ± 6.8	63.2 ± 6.7 **	TxS = 2.104	0.151	0.026
					TxBMI = 0.512	0.476	0.006
					TxC = 0.269	0.765	0.007
					TxSxBMIxC = 0.615	0.543	0.015
TEI (kcal)							
Baseline	2447.9 ± 1026.8	2434.3 ± 805.2	2766.2 ± 1186.0	2592.9 ± 1044.5	T = 41.841	<0.001	0.377
Post-intervention	1781.5 ± 448.5	1811.0 ± 563.9	1850.5 ± 651.7	1823.3 ± 580.4 **	TxS = 3.670	0.060	0.051
					TxBMI = 6.725	0.012	0.089
					TxC = 1.554	0.219	0.043
					TxSxBMIxC = 2.115	.128	0.058

Table 3. *Cont.*

	<7500	≥7500<10,000	≥10,000	Total	F	p	η_p^2
CHO (%)							
Baseline	38.5 ± 7.8	36.3 ± 7.0	37.8 ± 6.2	37.5 ± 6.8	T = 30.129	<0.001	0.304
Post-intervention	44.0 ± 6.1	43.2 ± 6.1	43.2 ± 6.3	43.4 ± 6.1 **	TxS = 1.698	0.197	0.024
					TxBMI = 0.531	0.469	0.008
					TxC = 0.559	0.575	0.016
					TxSxBMIxC = 0.985	0.379	0.028
PRO (%)							
Baseline	17.3 ± 3.5	17.6 ± 2.1	16.3 ± 2.5	16.9 ± 2.6	T = 36.812	<0.001	0.348
Post-intervention	19.1 ± 2.5	19.2 ± 2.5	20.3 ± 2.7	19.7 ± 2.6 **	TxS < 0.001	0.994	<0.001
					TxBMI = 1.440	0.234	0.020
					TxC = 4.587	0.013	0.117
					TxSxBMIxC = 0.962	0.387	0.027
FAT (%)							
Baseline	40.7 ± 7.9	41.5 ± 6.9	41.1 ± 6.1	41.2 ± 6.7	T = 48.246	<0.001	0.411
Post-intervention	33.4 ± 5.5	33.9 ± 6.0	33.4 ± 6.0	33.5 ± 5.8 **	TxS = 0.296	0.588	0.004
					TxBMI = 0.716	0.400	0.010
					TxC = 0.316	0.730	0.009
					TxSxBMIxC = 1.674	0.195	0.046
MOTIVATION TO DIET							
Baseline	70.0 ± 7.2	71.0 ± 6.9	70.9 ± 6.3	70.7 ± 6.6	T = 11.851	0.001	0.130
Post-intervention	73.1 ± 5.6	73.5 ± 6.4	72.2 ± 6.8	72.8 ± 6.4 *	TxS = 1.838	0.179	0.023
					TxBMI = 0.496	0.483	0.006
					TxC = 0.704	0.498	0.018
					TxSxBMIxC = 1.170	0.316	0.029
MOTIVATION TO EXERCISE							
Baseline	17.5 ± 3.6	18.4 ± 1.7	17.8 ± 2.4	18.0 ± 2.5	T = 1.422	0.237	0.018
Post-intervention	18.1 ± 4.5	18.2 ± 3.7	18.4 ± 2.2	18.3 ± 3.3	TxS = 6.305	0.014	0.074
					TxBMI = 2.325	0.131	0.029
					TxC = 0.494	0.612	0.012
					TxSxBMIxC = 0.609	0.546	0.015

TEI: total energy intake; CHO: carbohydrate intake; PRO: protein intake; FAT: fat intake; T: time (pre-post); S: gender; BMI: body mass index category; C: daily steps' categories. * $p < 0.05$; ** $p < 0.001$.

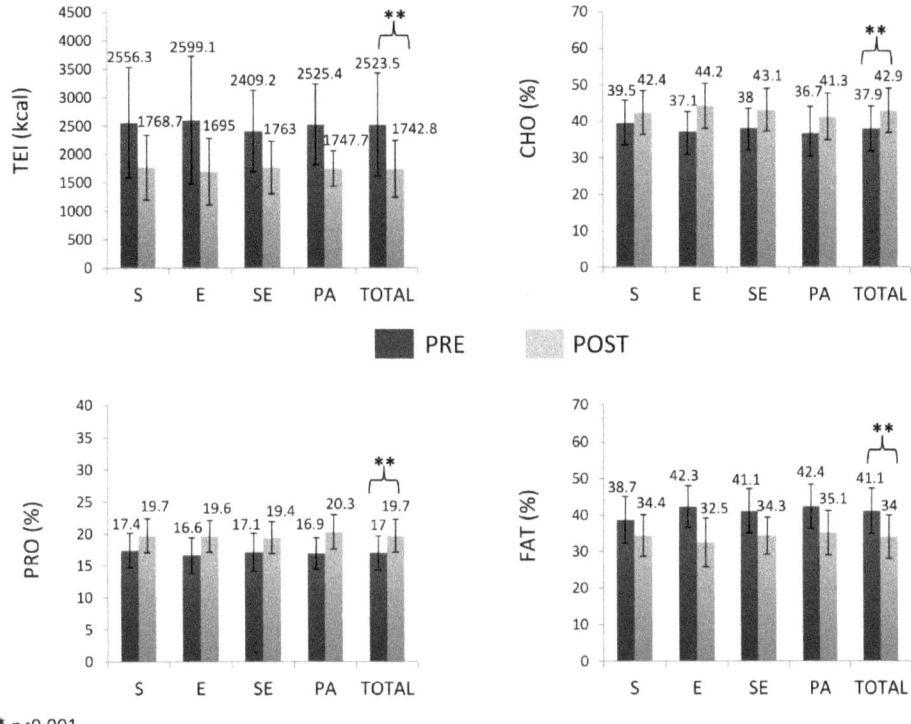

** *p*<0.001

Figure 3. Total energy intake and macronutrient percentages before and after the intervention. TEI: total energy intake; CHO: carbohydrate intake; PRO: protein intake; FAT: fat intake; S: strength training group; E: endurance training group; SE: combined strength plus endurance training group; PA: physical activity recommendations group.

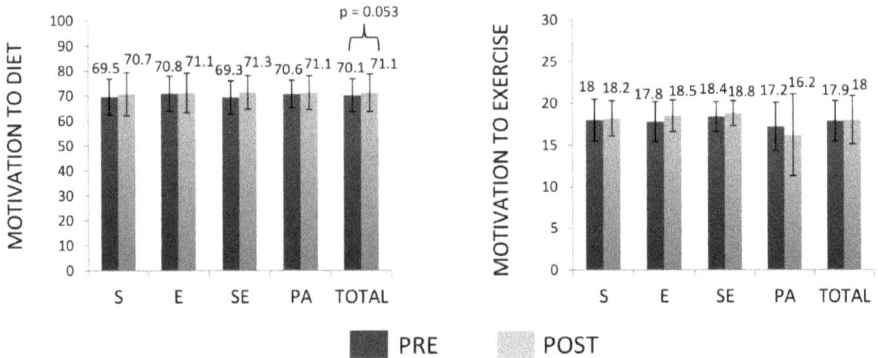

Figure 4. Motivation to diet and exercise before and after the intervention. S: strength training group; E: endurance training group; SE: strength and endurance training group; PA: physical activity recommendations group.

4. Discussion

The main findings of this study were: (1) Macronutrient distribution and total caloric intake did not differ among strength, endurance, combined or guideline-based physical activity groups; (2) if diet advices are included, long-term exercise programs do not increase energy intake in a compensatory fashion; (3) individuals that started the program performing >7500 daily steps revealed greater increases in protein intake; (4) motivation to exercise increased only in women.

To the best of our knowledge, this is the first study to investigate macronutrient distribution among three different types of exercise interventions in circuit. Our results are in accordance with previous findings that have suggested there is no substantial effect of a specific exercise on macronutrient selection [5,20]. The literature is limited and there are very few trials of sufficient duration [21]. A recent meta-analysis investigating whether an increase in exercise or physical activity could alter ad-libitum daily energy intake or macronutrient composition in healthy adults, evaluated 24 randomized trials. From these 24 trials, only two evaluated different types of exercise [21]. Shaw et al. [22] compared the effects of endurance and combined training in normal weight subjects, while Bales et al. [23], compared the effects of endurance, resistance and the linear combination of both in obese individuals. As in our study, their results also pointed to a reduction in energy intake; however these studies did not find any change in the percentage contribution of each macronutrient.

Our data showed similar decreases in fat intake in all intervention groups. Many studies found consistent negative associations between fat intake and BMI or waist circumference, besides pointing to a contribution of diet composition, especially saturated fat and refined carbohydrates, in oxidative stress and inflammation [24]. Thus, decreases, observed in this study for fat intake, could contribute to a healthier life, considering that the Spanish population typically presents an excessive consumption of fats [25]. Our results also showed an increase of CHO and PRO intakes in all intervention groups. This homogeneous change among the four groups in our study could be due to the fact that all individuals received the same diet restriction and advices, which probably influenced these responses. Other factors, as exercise intensity [9], genetics [26], or social conditions [27], also could induce differences in macronutrient selection. Furthermore, conscious food choices could mask the exercise effects to consume a particular combination of macronutrients [5].

A significant decrease in the total energy intake in response to all interventions was observed in our study, demonstrating that various types of exercise and physical activity recommendations, allied to diet, can be effective in maintaining lower energy intake even after the end of the program. The energy deficits achieved in this study (about 780 kcal) can be considered clinically meaningful and relevant for weight management, since a deficit of 100 kcal and 189 kcal per day have been estimated to prevent weight regain [28]. Our results confirmed the claim that sedentary individuals who initiate a long-term exercise program do not increase their energy intake in a compensatory fashion [23], if diet advices are included.

In our study, although the sample was sedentary at the beginning of the intervention (<30 min physical activity/day), subjects who started the program with more daily steps presented an increase in protein intake, although diet recommendations were equal for all the participants. Other studies have shown that active individuals consumed more protein than inactive counterparts [10,29]. This fact could be related to the belief that active individuals need to consume more proteins than sedentary individuals [10].

Regarding motivation to diet and exercise, our findings indicated a good acceptance of the intervention program by the individuals. Although, motivation to exercise increased only in women, men did not decrease it. These findings are in line with previous studies observing differences in motivation to exercise between men and women [30]. According to this study, the reasons for exercise seem to differ between genders, with men being more motivated by competitiveness and exceeding limits, while women tend to be more motivated by aspects related to aesthetics [31]. Still, prior research has shown that better quality motivations for exercise (i.e., autonomous) can be effectively promoted in weight management interventions, contributing to sustained weight loss [32]. Weman-Josefsson et al. [33], showed that exercise autonomous (i.e., good quality) motivation was a stronger predictor of continued exercise participation for women rather than for men. Therefore, in our study, weight loss could have contributed for an increase in autonomous motivation in women. Future studies should confirm this hypothesis.

Nutritional education alone may not be sufficient for changing eating behavior [34], and variations in adopted behaviors can affect energy balance and weight loss success. In this sense, exercise seems to play an important role in inducing better energy deficit in relation to dietary restriction, through the prevention of nutritional compensatory responses [35]. Furthermore, a strong relationship between exercise and eating behavior has been observed, and individuals who reported being internally motivated to eat were significantly more likely to engage in physical activity and presented lower BMI [36,37]. In fact, studies have indicated that emotionally-driven eating was related with less engagement in physical activity [38] and higher BMI [39,40].

Although ANOVA has not showed differences among intervention groups in energy intake, macronutrient distribution or motivations to diet and to exercise, some correlation results are worth to be commented upon. Correlations between motivations to diet and to exercise were found for all groups, except for the strength group. In general, the correlations observed in the strength group showed that individuals who ate more also moved more, and those who ate less moved less. The strength group was the only one that, although not significantly, increased absolute lean mass (data not shown). Blundell et al. [41] observed that fat-free mass was positively associated with daily energy intake and hunger levels, which could explain, at least in part, some results found in this group. Guelfi and colleagues [42] found that aerobic exercise was associated with an increase in satiety, while an equivalent period of 12 weeks of resistance training was not. It is possible that resistance exercise needs more time to improve the responses related to appetite control and further research should investigate these responses in relation to chronic exercise in a longer period of time (one year or more).

Nutritional behavior plays an important role in predicting cardiovascular risk for any category of BMI, and exercise behavior is also an important predictor for the presence of normal weight or overweight [43]. Further research is required to determine the mechanisms through which exercise training may affect and improve eating behavior, besides increasing the understanding that obesity is not a simple matter of will power or that merely eating less and exercising more is the solution [44]. Desirable eating and physical activity habits can be the best allies against overweight and its consequences, without adverse effects, unlike other methods such as herbal weight-loss products [45] or medications [46]. Success in long-term weight loss and maintenance increases as more behavioral dimensions are involved in the behavior change process [47].

There are many strengths in the study, such as the randomized design; inclusion of four different training programs in the same study, combined with caloric restriction in all interventions, and inclusion of appropriate programs of strength and combined training for comparison among groups, however, some limitations can be highlighted, including; [1] non-assessment behavioral/psychological markers of eating behavior (food cravings, emotional eating, eating disinhibition, etc.); [2] non-inclusion of a 'no treatment' control group; but rather compared the new intervention with the previous one that has been proven to be effective (i.e., diet and exercise recommendations) and is broadly accepted from an ethical point of view and in clinical practice; [3] non-compliance with the criteria for the analysis of the accelerometry data pointed to the difficulty of the use of the equipment by the subjects, and did not allow a more complete analysis of the data to be performed.

5. Conclusions

In conclusion, individuals who initiate a long-term exercise program do not increase their energy intake in a compensatory fashion, if diet advices are included. Our findings suggest that there is no substantial effect of the type of exercise on macronutrient selection or energy intake, but they point out a general change on these parameters when an exercise program is followed. Significant increases in carbohydrate and protein intakes and decreases in fat and total energy intakes were reported, regardless of the type of exercise, BMI category or gender, as a result of following a weight loss program. Furthermore, in a subsample of the present study, individuals who started the intervention performing higher number of daily steps increased more their protein intake than those who performed <7500 daily steps. Lastly, there were increases in diet and exercise motivations, although motivation to exercise was incremented only in women.

Author Contributions: The study was designed by D.G.-L., E.A.C. and E.V.C.; data were collected and analyzed by A.B.P., B.L.-P., E.A.C., E.V.C and R.C.; data interpretation and manuscript preparation were undertaken by A.B.P., B.L.-P., D.G.-L., E.A.C., E.V.C., P.J.T. and R.C. All authors have read and agreed to the published version of the manuscript.

Funding: The PRONAF Study takes place with the financial support of the Ministerio de Ciencia e Innovación, Convocatoria de Ayudas I+D 2008, Proyectos de Investigación Fundamental No Orientada, del VI Plan de Investigación Nacional 2008-2011, (Contract: DEP2008-06354-C04-01). This study was financed in part by the Coordenação de Aperfeiçoamento de Pessoal de Nível Superior—Brasil (CAPES)—Finance Code 001.

Acknowledgments: We thank to the participants and professionals involved in this study.

Conflicts of Interest: The authors declare no conflict of interest.

References

1. Global Burden of Metabolic Risk Factors for Chronic Diseases Collaboration (BMI Mediated Effects); Lu, Y.; Hajifathalian, K.; Ezzati, M.; Woodward, M.; Rimm, E.B.; Danaei, G. Metabolic mediators of the effects of body-mass index, overweight, and obesity on coronary heart disease and stroke: A pooled analysis of 97 prospective cohorts with 1·8 million participants. *Lancet* **2014**, *383*, 970–983. [CrossRef]
2. Dombrowski, S.U.; Knittle, K.; Avenell, A.; Araújo-Soares, V.; Sniehotta, F.F. Long term maintenance of weight loss with non-surgical interventions in obese adults: Systematic review and meta-analyses of randomised controlled trials. *BMJ* **2014**, *348*, g2646. [CrossRef]
3. Fisher, G.; Hyatt, T.C.; Hunter, G.R.; Oster, R.A.; Desmond, R.A.; Gower, B.A. Effect of diet with and without exercise training on markers of inflammation and fat distribution in overweight women. *Obesity* **2011**, *19*, 1131–1136. [CrossRef]
4. Blundell, J.E.; Gibbons, C.; Caudwell, P.; Finlayson, G.; Hopkins, M. Appetite control and energy balance: Impact of exercise. *Obes. Rev.* **2015**, *16* (Suppl. 1), 67–76. [CrossRef]
5. Elder, S.J.; Roberts, S.B. The effects of exercise on food intake and body fatness: A summary of published studies. *Nutr. Rev.* **2007**, *65*, 1–19. [CrossRef]
6. Schubert, M.M.; Sabapathy, S.; Leveritt, M.; Desbrow, B. Acute exercise and hormones related to appetite regulation: A meta-analysis. *Sports Med.* **2014**, *44*, 387–403. [CrossRef]
7. Martins, C.; Kulseng, B.; King, N.A.; Holst, J.J.; Blundell, J.E. The effects of exercise-induced weight loss on appetite-related peptides and motivation to eat. *J. Clin. Endocrinol. Metab.* **2010**, *95*, 1609–1616. [CrossRef]
8. Whybrow, S.; Hughes, D.A.; Ritz, P.; Johnstone, A.M.; Horgan, G.W.; King, N.; Blundell, J.E.; Stubbs, R.J. The effect of an incremental increase in exercise on appetite, eating behaviour and energy balance in lean men and women feeding ad libitum. *Br. J. Nutr.* **2008**, *100*, 1109–1115. [CrossRef]
9. Alkahtani, S.A.; Byrne, N.M.; Hills, A.P.; King, N.A. Interval training intensity affects energy intake compensation in obese men. *Int. J. Sport Nutr. Exerc. Metab.* **2014**, *24*, 595–604. [CrossRef]
10. Jokisch, E.; Coletta, A.; Raynor, H.A. Acute energy compensation and macronutrient intake following exercise in active and inactive males who are normal weight. *Appetite* **2012**, *58*, 722–729. [CrossRef]
11. Carraça, E.V.; Silva, M.N.; Coutinho, S.R.; Vieira, P.N.; Minderico, C.S.; Sardinha, L.B.; Teixeira, P.J. The association between physical activity and eating self-regulation in overweight and obese women. *Obes. Facts* **2013**, *6*, 493–506. [CrossRef] [PubMed]
12. Lowe, C.J.; Hall, P.A.; Vincent, C.M.; Luu, K. The effects of acute aerobic activity on cognition and cross-domain transfer to eating behavior. *Front. Hum. Neurosci.* **2014**, *8*, 267. [CrossRef] [PubMed]
13. Zapico, A.G.; Benito, P.J.; González-Gross, M.; Peinado, A.B.; Morencos, E.; Romero, B.; Rojo-Tirado, M.A.; Cupeiro, R.; Szendrei, B.; Butragueño, J.; et al. Nutrition and physical activity programs for obesity treatment (PRONAF study): Methodological approach of the project. *BMC Public Health* **2012**, *12*, 1100. [CrossRef] [PubMed]

14. Donnelly, J.E.; Blair, S.N.; Jakicic, J.M.; Manore, M.M.; Rankin, J.W.; Smith, B.K. American College of Sports Medicine. American College of Sports Medicine Position Stand. Appropriate physical activity intervention strategies for weight loss and prevention of weight regain for adults. *Med. Sci. Sports Exerc.* **2009**, *41*, 459–471. [CrossRef]

15. Serra-Majem, L.; Aranceta, J.; SENC Working Group on Nutritional Objectives for the Spanish Population. Spanish Society of Community Nutrition. Nutritional objectives for the Spanish population. Consensus from the Spanish Society of Community Nutrition. *Public Health Nutr.* **2001**, *4*, 1409–1413. [CrossRef]

16. Castro, E.A.; Júdice, P.B.; Silva, A.M.; Teixeira, P.J.; Benito, P.J. Sedentary behavior and compensatory mechanisms in response to different doses of exercise—A randomized controlled trial in overweight and obese adults. *Eur. J. Clin. Nutr.* **2017**, *71*, 1393–1398. [CrossRef]

17. Tudor-Locke, C.; Craig, C.L.; Brown, W.J.; Clemes, S.A.; De Cocker, K.; Giles-Corti, B.; Hatano, Y.; Inoue, S.; Matsudo, S.M.; Mutrie, N.; et al. How many steps/day are enough? For adults. *Int. J. Behav. Nutr. Phys. Act.* **2011**, *8*, 79. [CrossRef]

18. Ortega, R.; Requejo, A.; Lopez-Sobaler, A. Questionniares for dietetic studies and the assessment of nutritional status. In *Nutriguía Manual of Clinical Nutrition in Primary Care*; Requejo, A., Ortega, R., Eds.; Editorial Complutense: Madrid, Spain, 2003.

19. Richardson, J.T. Eta squared and partial eta squared as measures of effect size in educational research. *Educ. Res. Rev.* **2011**, *6*, 135–147. [CrossRef]

20. Washburn, R.A.; Honas, J.J.; Ptomey, L.T.; Mayo, M.S.; Lee, J.; Sullivan, D.K.; Lambourne, K.; Willis, E.A.; Donnelly, J.E. Energy and Macronutrient Intake in the Midwest Exercise Trial 2 (MET-2). *Med. Sci. Sports Exerc.* **2015**, *47*, 1941–1949. [CrossRef]

21. Donnelly, J.E.; Herrmann, S.D.; Lambourne, K.; Szabo, A.N.; Honas, J.J.; Washburn, R.A. Does increased exercise or physical activity alter ad-libitum daily energy intake or macronutrient composition in healthy adults? A systematic review. *PLoS ONE* **2014**, *9*, e83498. [CrossRef]

22. Shaw, B.S.; Shaw, I.; Mamen, A. Contrasting effects in anthropometric measures of total fatness and abdominal fat mass following endurance and concurrent endurance and resistance training. *J. Sports Med. Phys. Fit.* **2010**, *50*, 207–213.

23. Bales, C.W.; Hawk, V.H.; Granville, E.O.; Rose, S.B.; Shields, T.; Bateman, L.; Willis, L.; Piner, L.W.; Slentz, C.A.; Houmard, J.A.; et al. Aerobic and resistance training effects on energy intake: The STRRIDE-AT/RT study. *Med. Sci. Sports Exerc.* **2012**, *44*, 2033–2039. [CrossRef] [PubMed]

24. Dandona, P.; Ghanim, H.; Chaudhuri, A.; Dhindsa, S.; Kim, S.S. Macronutrient intake induces oxidative and inflammatory stress: Potential relevance to atherosclerosis and insulin resistance. *Exp. Mol. Med.* **2010**, *42*, 245–253. [CrossRef] [PubMed]

25. González-Solanellas, M.; Romagosa Pérez-Portabella, A.; Zabaleta-Del-Olmo, E.; Grau-Carod, M.; Casellas-Montagut, C.; Lancho-Lancho, S.; Moreno-Feliu, R.; Pérez-Portabella, M.C. Prevalence of food habits and nutritional status in adult population served in primary care. *Nutr. Hosp.* **2011**, *26*, 337–344. [CrossRef] [PubMed]

26. Goni, L.; Cuervo, M.; Milagro, F.I.; Martínez, J.A. A genetic risk tool for obesity predisposition assessment and personalized nutrition implementation based on macronutrient intake. *Genes. Nutr.* **2015**, *10*, 445. [CrossRef]

27. Riesco, E.; Tessier, S.; Pérusse, F.; Turgeon, S.; Tremblay, A.; Weisnagel, J.; Doré, J.; Mauriège, P. Impact of walking on eating behaviors and quality of life of premenopausal and early postmenopausal obese women. *Menopause* **2010**, *17*, 529–538. [CrossRef]

28. Sim, A.Y.; Wallman, K.E.; Fairchild, T.J.; Guelfi, K.J. Effects of High-Intensity Intermittent Exercise Training on Appetite Regulation. *Med. Sci. Sports Exerc.* **2015**, *47*, 2441–2449. [CrossRef]

29. Varlet-Marie, E.; Guiraudou, M.; Fédou, C.; Raynaud de Mauverger, E.; Durand, F.; Brun, J.F. Nutritional and metabolic determinants of blood rheology differ between trained and sedentary individuals. *Clin. Hemorheol. Microcirc.* **2013**, *55*, 39–54. [CrossRef]

30. San Mauro Martín, I.; Garicano Vilar, E.; González Fernández, M.; Villacorta Pérez, P.; Megias Gamarra, A.; Miralles Rivera, B.; Figueroa Borque, M.; Andrés Sánchez, N.; Bonilla Navarro, M.Á.; Arranz Poza, P.; et al. Nutritional and psychological habits in people who practice exercise. *Nutr. Hosp.* **2014**, *30*, 1324–1332. [CrossRef]

31. Balbinotti, M.A.A.; Capozzoli, C.J. [Motivação à prática regular de atividade física: Um estudo exploratório com praticantes em academias de ginástica]. Rev. bras. *Educ. Fís. Esp.* **2008**, *22*, 63–80. [CrossRef]
32. Silva, M.N.; Markland, D.; Carraça, E.V.; Vieira, P.N.; Coutinho, S.R.; Minderico, C.S.; Matos, M.G.; Sardinha, L.B.; Teixeira, P.J. Exercise autonomous motivation predicts 3-yr weight loss in women. *Med. Sci. Sports Exerc.* **2011**, *43*, 728–737. [CrossRef] [PubMed]
33. Weman-Josefsson, K.; Lindwall, M.; Ivarsson, A. Need satisfaction, motivational regulations and exercise: Moderation and mediation effects. *Int. J. Behav. Nutr. Phys. Act.* **2015**, *12*, 67. [CrossRef] [PubMed]
34. Annesi, J.J.; Walsh, A.M.; Smith, A.E. Effects of 12- and 24-week multimodal interventions on physical activity, nutritional behaviors, and body mass index and its psychological predictors in severely obese adolescents at risk for diabetes. *Perm. J.* **2010**, *14*, 29–37. [CrossRef] [PubMed]
35. Thivel, D.; Doucet, E.; Julian, V.; Cardenoux, C.; Boirie, Y.; Duclos, M. Nutritional compensation to exercise- vs. diet-induced acute energy deficit in adolescents with obesity. *Physiol. Behav.* **2017**, *176*, 159–164. [CrossRef]
36. Cadena-Schlam, L.; López-Guimerà, G. Intuitive eating: An emerging approach to eating behavior. *Nutr. Hosp.* **2014**, *31*, 995–1002. [CrossRef] [PubMed]
37. Gast, J.; Campbell Nielson, A.; Hunt, A.; Leiker, J.J. Intuitive eating: Associations with physical activity motivation and BMI. *Am. J. Health Promot.* **2015**, *29*, e91–e99. [CrossRef]
38. Whitaker, K.M.; Sharpe, P.A.; Wilcox, S.; Hutto, B.E. Depressive symptoms are associated with dietary intake but not physical activity among overweight and obese women from disadvantaged neighborhoods. *Nutr. Res.* **2014**, *34*, 294–301. [CrossRef]
39. Danielsen, K.K.; Svendsen, M.; Mæhlum, S.; Sundgot-Borgen, J. Changes in body composition, cardiovascular disease risk factors, and eating behavior after an intensive lifestyle intervention with high volume of physical activity in severely obese subjects: A prospective clinical controlled trial. *J. Obes.* **2013**, *2013*, 325464. [CrossRef]
40. Stein, K.F.; Chen, D.G.; Corte, C.; Keller, C.; Trabold, N. Disordered eating behaviors in young adult Mexican American women: Prevalence and associations with health risks. *Eat. Behav.* **2013**, *14*, 476–483. [CrossRef]
41. Blundell, J.E.; Caudwell, P.; Gibbons, C.; Hopkins, M.; Naslund, E.; King, N.; Finlayson, G. Role of resting metabolic rate and energy expenditure in hunger and appetite control: A new formulation. *Dis. Model. Mech.* **2012**, *5*, 608–613. [CrossRef]
42. Guelfi, K.J.; Donges, C.E.; Duffield, R. Beneficial effects of 12 weeks of aerobic compared with resistance exercise training on perceived appetite in previously sedentary overweight and obese men. *Metabolism* **2013**, *62*, 235–243. [CrossRef] [PubMed]
43. Huang, J.H.; Huang, S.L.; Li, R.H.; Wang, L.H.; Chen, Y.L.; Tang, F.C. Effects of nutrition and exercise health behaviors on predicted risk of cardiovascular disease among workers with different body mass index levels. *Int. J. Environ. Res. Public Health* **2014**, *11*, 4664–4675. [CrossRef] [PubMed]
44. Brown, R.E.; Sharma, A.M.; Ardern, C.I.; Mirdamadi, P.; Mirdamadi, P.; Kuk, J.L. Secular differences in the association between caloric intake, macronutrient intake, and physical activity with obesity. *Obes. Res. Clin. Pract.* **2016**, *10*, 359–360. [CrossRef] [PubMed]
45. Bersani, F.S.; Coviello, M.; Imperatori, C.; Francesconi, M.; Hough, C.M.; Valeriani, G.; De Stefano, G.; Bolzan Mariotti Posocco, F.; Santacroce, R.; Minichino, A.; et al. Adverse psychiatric effects associated with herbal weight-loss products. *Biomed. Res. Int.* **2015**. [CrossRef]
46. Khera, R.; Murad, M.H.; Chandar, A.K.; Dulai, P.S.; Wang, Z.; Prokop, L.J.; Loomba, R.; Camilleri, M.; Singh, S. Association of pharmacological treatments for obesity with weight loss and adverse events: A systematic review and meta-analysis. *JAMA* **2016**, *315*, 2424–2434. [CrossRef]
47. Westenhoefer, J. The therapeutic challenge: Behavioral changes for long-term weight maintenance. *Int. J. Obes. Relat. Metab. Disord.* **2001**, *25* (Suppl. 1), S85–S88. [CrossRef]

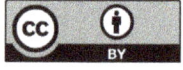

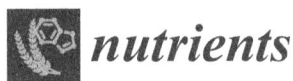

Article

The Impact of Coconut Oil and Epigallocatechin Gallate on the Levels of IL-6, Anxiety and Disability in Multiple Sclerosis Patients

Jose Luis Platero [1], María Cuerda-Ballester [2], Vanessa Ibáñez [2], David Sancho [2], María Mar Lopez-Rodríguez [3,*], Eraci Drehmer [4] and Jose Enrique de la Rubia Ortí [2]

[1] Doctoral Degree School, Catholic University of Valencia San Vicente Martir, 46001 Valencia, Spain; joseluisplateroarmero@gmail.com

[2] Department of Nursing, Catholic University of Valencia San Vicente Martir, 46001 Valencia, Spain; m.cuerda@hotmail.com (M.C.-B.); vanessa.ibanez@ucv.es (V.I.); david.sancho@ucv.es (D.S.); joseenrique.delarubi@ucv.es (J.E.d.l.R.O.)

[3] Department of Nursing, Physiotherapy and Medicine, University of Almería, 04120 Almería, Spain

[4] Department of Physical Activity and Sport Sciences, Catholic University of Valencia San Vicente Martir, 46001 Valencia, Spain; eraci.drehmer@ucv.es

* Correspondence: mlr295@ual.es; Tel.: +34-95-0015374

Received: 19 December 2019; Accepted: 19 January 2020; Published: 23 January 2020

Abstract: Background: Due to the inflammatory nature of multiple sclerosis (MS), interleukin 6 (IL-6) is high in blood levels, and it also increases the levels of anxiety related to functional disability. Epigallocatechin gallate (EGCG) decreases IL-6, which could be enhanced by the anti-inflammatory effect of high ketone bodies after administering coconut oil (both of which are an anxiolytic). Therefore, the aim of this study was to assess the impact of coconut oil and EGCG on the levels of IL-6, anxiety and functional disability in patients with MS. Methods: A pilot study was conducted for four months with 51 MS patients who were randomly divided into an intervention group and a control group. The intervention group received 800 mg of EGCG and 60 mL of coconut oil, and the control group was prescribed a placebo. Both groups followed the same isocaloric Mediterranean diet. State and trait anxiety were determined before and after the study by means of the State-Trait Anxiety Inventory (STAI). In addition, IL-6 in serum was measured using the ELISA technique and functional capacity was determined with the Expanded Disability Status Scale (EDSS) and the body mass index (BMI). Results: State anxiety and functional capacity decreased in the intervention group and IL-6 decreased in both groups. Conclusions: EGCG and coconut oil improve state anxiety and functional capacity. In addition, a decrease in IL-6 is observed in patients with MS, possibly due to the antioxidant capacity of the Mediterranean diet and its impact on improving BMI.

Keywords: multiple sclerosis; epigallocatechin gallate; coconut oil; interleukin-6; anxiety; disability

---

1. Introduction

Multiple sclerosis (MS) is a chronic, inflammatory and autoimmune disease of the central nervous system (CNS) that causes a progressive deterioration of the myelin sheath associated with axonal injuries at a neuronal level, leading to functional disability. This neuronal damage is mainly based on high oxidative stress and inflammation in the central nervous system, affecting the permeability of the blood–brain barrier (BBB) and allowing autoreactive T cells, B cells, macrophages and microglia to access and especially damage the white matter in the brain and spinal cord [1–3].

Due to the inflammatory nature of MS, several inflammatory markers have been related to the disease, especially interleukin 6 (IL-6) whose levels are significantly high in MS patients [4]. Thus, it has been demonstrated that T cells in MS patients have more IL-6 receptors in peripheral blood than healthy individuals [5]. Due to the fact that it is an inflammatory marker, the amounts increase when the person is overweight or obese, which is determined by means of anthropometric parameters, such as the body mass index (BMI) [6] that is correlated with the individual's adiposity [7]. Clinically speaking, there is a relation to characteristic aspects of the disease, such as relapses and functional disability [4], and with its pathogenesis [8].

Nonetheless, patients with a higher concentration of IL-6 in serum show higher levels of anxiety [9]. Thus, the most anxious individuals have higher levels of IL-6, regardless of their age or gender [10]. Anxiety has been observed to influence the level of inflammation, increasing the risk of developing inflammatory diseases [11]. The influence of anxiety is due to a transcriptional pattern observed in animal models, in which monocytes are recruited that specifically depend on the increase of IL-6 in serum [12], once anxiety in stressful situations is caused. As a result of this link between the high levels of IL-6 and the perception of anxiety, we can see that anxiety disorders are found amongst the most common psychiatric disorders associated with MS [13]. In addition, anxiety symptoms have an effect on the course of the disease, increasing the levels of fatigue [14] and especially functional disability [15].

In this sense, ketone bodies obtained through hepatic beta-oxidation have shown improvements in inflammatory markers, including lipid markers, glycated haemoglobin (HbA1c) or high-sensitivity C-reactive proteins that are related to an increase in the total antioxidant state in blood [16]. Particularly in MS, the ketone body β-hydroxybutyrate (BHB) activates HCA2 receptors expressed by neuroinflammatory cells, reducing neuroinflammation [17] and achieving a neuroprotective effect [18]. In addition, ketone bodies have decreased the perception of anxiety in animal models with Alzheimer's disease, where an anxiolytic effect of the ketogenic diet has been observed [19], and in humans of advanced age [20]. Regarding the nutrients capable of providing higher levels of ketone bodies in blood, those with high levels of medium-chain triglycerides (MCTs) stand out, with coconut oil possibly being the food with the highest amount of MCTs, due to the high percentages of medium-chain fatty acids (MCFAs), such as lauric acid, palmitic acid, stearic acid, myristic acid and oleic acid [21]. These acids are absorbed intact and do not suffer degradation and reesterification processes [22].

On the other hand, epigallocatechin gallate (EGCG) is a polyphenolic catechin with a high antioxidant and anti-inflammatory activity [23,24]. EGCG's protective effect allows it to be especially efficient in autoimmune diseases, such as MS, as it promotes the repression of autoreactive T cell proliferation, a reduced production of proinflammatory cytokines, a decrease in Th1 and Th17, as well as an increase in the regulatory T cell populations in lymphoid tissues and the CNS [25]. It also takes the spotlight due to its capacity to penetrate the blood–brain barrier [26] and to accumulate inside the mitochondria of the neurons, decreasing apoptosis due to the high oxidative stress of the disease [27].

Finally, EGCG is also related to an emotional improvement, especially in terms of anxiety, as the activity of GABA receptors is modulated [28]. This would explain the decrease in anxiety after administration in CNS diseases, such as schizophrenia [29]. Therefore, the aim of this study was to assess the impact of coconut oil and EGCG on the levels of IL-6 and anxiety related to functional disability in MS patients.

2. Materials and Methods

A prospective, mixed and experimental pilot study was conducted by means of a clinical trial.

2.1. Subjects

The population sample was obtained from the main state-wide MS associations who were previously informed on the characteristics of the study. Sixty-seven people were interested in voluntarily taking part in the study. The following selection criteria were applied: patients over 18 years of age diagnosed with MS at least 6 months prior and treated with glatiramer acetate and interferon beta. On the other hand, the exclusion criteria included: pregnant or breastfeeding women, patients with tracheotomy, stoma or with short bowel syndrome, patients with dementia, evidence of alcohol or drug abuse, with myocardial infarction, heart failure, cardia dysrhythmia, symptoms of angina or other heart conditions, patients with kidney conditions with creatinine levels two times higher than normal markers, patients with elevated liver markers three times higher than normal or with chronic liver disease, patients with metabolic or endocrine diseases such as hyperthyroidism or diabetes, patients with acromegaly, patients with polycystic ovary syndrome or MS patients who were included in other researches with experimental drugs or treatment.

2.2. Statistical Analysis

Statistical analysis was performed with the SPSS v.23 (IBM Corporation, Armonk, NY, USA) tool. The first step aimed to estimate the distribution of the variables investigated through statistical methods to assess normality, including the Kolmogorov–Smirnov Test. This analysis demonstrated the non-normal distribution of all the scale variables studied. Therefore, the U de Mann–Whitney test and the Wilcoxon signed-rank test were used to assess the inter-group and pre-post differences, respectively. Categorical data were analysed with a chi-square test. A p-value below 0.05 was considered significant. Data are presented as mean ± standard deviation, or the number of patients and percentage.

2.3. Procedure

Once the final population sample was obtained, the patients received further information on the study, as well as the set objectives and the tests and analyses that would be carried out. They were also provided with instructions to not change the prescribed diet for each case (depending on whether they were in the control group or intervention group), as well as to take the capsules on a daily basis at the scheduled times over the 4-month duration of the intervention. In order to verify the patients complied with the treatment, members of the team made weekly telephone calls (on Monday mornings) to each and every patient. They were asked about any doubts or incidences regarding the diet, with the aim of ensuring the caloric intake was followed, or whether they had had any issue with the capsules (such as an intolerance or side effect). These calls were carried out over the 4 months of the duration of the intervention. No general issues or problems with the diet or capsules were registered.

2.4. Intervention

Once the selection criteria had been applied, a final sample of 51 MS patients was obtained. They were randomly divided into the intervention and control group. The intervention group received an isocaloric diet for 4 months (adapted to the individual characteristics of each patient and divided into 5 meals a day: breakfast, mid-morning snack, lunch, afternoon snack and dinner) enriched with 60 mL of extra virgin coconut oil divided into 2 equal intakes (30 mL for breakfast and 30 mL for lunch), and supplemented with 800 mg of EGCG administered in two capsules of 400 mg to be taken twice a day (once capsule in the morning and another in the afternoon).

On the other hand, the control group followed the same isocaloric diet as the intervention group for the same 4 months, as well as administering placebo (capsules containing microcrystalline cellulose, matching in size and colour). They followed the same instructions as the intervention group. The base diet followed by both groups included the following percentage distribution of the 3 main macronutrients with respect to the total caloric value: 20% proteins, 40% carbohydrates and 40% Mediterranean lipids.

This diet was based on the Mediterranean-type food pattern, and was characterised for being balanced, varied and with sufficient calories, by providing adequate food proportions divided into 5 daily intakes. The consumption of proteins with a high biological value of animal origin such as fresh fish, eggs and dairy products (milk, yoghurt and cheese) were highlighted, to the detriment of meat and meat products. In addition, plant protein was provided based on a combination of cereals and pulses. In terms of carbohydrates, they were complex and rich in fibre, provided from rice, cereals, wholegrain bread, pulses, tubers, vegetables and fruit. Regarding lipids, there was a predomination of monounsaturated fatty acids from extra virgin olive oil and nuts rich in omega-3 and omega-6, thus minimising the intake of saturated fatty acids. It is also important to highlight the high level of antioxidants in the diet, especially polyphenols estimated from the work carried out by Manach et al. [30] of 758.85 mg per day, per kg of various fresh foods containing them.

2.5. Measurements

The following measurements were taken before and after the 4-month intervention, in the same conditions and at the same time. In the specific case of the scales, they were carried out by the same neurologist assigned to each patient before the study.

2.5.1. State-Trait Anxiety Inventory (STAI)

This scale, used in clinical settings to diagnose anxiety and distinguish it from symptoms of depression [31], was published by Spielberger et al. [32] and validated for the Spanish population [33]. It is commonly used to obtain a significant measurement of state anxiety and trait anxiety. State anxiety refers to how the subject feels in a specific moment, while trait anxiety is described as how the individual normally feels. The inventory is made up of 40 questions, 20 about trait anxiety and 20 about state anxiety. All of the questions are given a 4-point frequency scale. The higher the points, the higher the perceived anxiety.

2.5.2. Expanded Disability Status Scale (EDSS)

This scale is used to assess functional disability in multiple sclerosis patients [34]. The scale is an ordinal scale based on a neurological examination of the eight functional systems (pyramidal, cerebellar, brainstem, mental, sensory, visual, bowel and bladder), alongside an assessment on walking capacity, which, as a result, provides a disability index between 0 and 10, 0 being understood as having normal health and 10 death by MS.

2.5.3. Blood Test and IL-6 Analysis

Blood tests were carried out in the peripheral vein (antecubital vein) at 11 a.m. on an empty stomach. The blood samples were collected in BD Vacutainer Plus serum blood collection tubes (ref. 367815). Once the test was finished, the samples were left at room temperature for 30 min to coagulate. The coagulated part was separated by centrifuging the samples at 4000 rounds/min for 10 min in a refrigerated centrifuge. After centrifuging, the supernatant liquid (blood serum) was transferred to 0.5 mL aliquots, which were then frozen and stored at -80 °C. Finally, the concentration of IL-6 in serum was determined after 24 h had passed. In order to do so, the aliquots were thawed and the ELISA technique (R&D Systems) was used.

2.5.4. Body Mass Index (BMI)

The body mass index is calculated as weight (kg)/height (m^2). Body weight was measured while the patient was wearing light clothes, no shoes and using a medical scale with a 0.5 kg precision. Height was measured with each patient standing up and using a medical tape measure with a 1 cm precision.

2.6. Ethical Concerns

The study was conducted in accordance with the Helsinki Declaration [35], prior approval of the protocol by the Human Research Committee of the University of Valencia of the Experimental Research Ethics Committee (procedure number H1512345043343). In addition, patients included in the study signed a consent form after being informed on the procedures and nature of the study.

3. Results

This study analysed a sample of 51 MS patients, divided into an intervention group and a control group, whose socio-demographic and clinical characteristics are shown in Table 1.

Table 1. Socio-demographic and clinical characteristics of the population of the study.

Measure		Group						p
		CG N = 24		IG N = 27		Total N = 51		
		Count	%	Count	%	Count	%	
MS type	Relapsing-Remitting	17	70.8%	20	74.1%	37	72.5%	0.796
	Secondary-Progressive	7	29.2%	7	25.9%	14	27.5%	
Gender	Man	10	41.7%	5	18.5%	15	29.4%	0.070
	Woman	14	58.3%	22	81.5%	36	70.6%	
Measure		Median	Range	Median	Range	Median	Range	p
Age (years)		50.50	45.00	45.00	48.00	47.00	48.00	0.119
Time since diagnosis (years)		13.50	35.00	9.00	35.00	12.00	37.00	0.156
IL-6 pre-test (pg/mL)		2.69	9.98	2.18	16.27	2.54	16.27	0.481
IL-6 post-test (pg/mL)		0.94	3.89	0.84	9.80	0.86	9.86	0.380
STAI state pre-test		19.50	29.00	23.00	38.00	22.00	38.00	0.720
STAI state post-test		20.00	33.00	17.00	34.00	19.00	36.00	0.242
STAI trait pre-test		24.50	42.00	32.00	49.00	28.00	51.00	0.223
STAI trait post-test		23.50	54.00	28.00	54.00	24.00	57.00	0.741
EDSS pre-test		3.75	6.50	3.00	6.50	3.50	6.50	0.435
EDSS post-test		3.75	6.50	3.00	5.50	3.50	6.50	0.351
BMI pre-test (kg/m^2)		24.61	23.17	23.43	19.09	24.24	23.17	0.992
BMI post-test (kg/m^2)		23.54	21.74	23.49	18.05	23.54	21.74	0.946

Z: U de Mann Whitney; CG: control group; IG: intervention group; MS: multiple sclerosis; EDSS: Expanded Disability Status Scale; IL-6: interleukin 6; STAI: State-Trait Anxiety Inventory; BMI: body mass index; SD: standard deviation.

After the 4-month intervention, the changes in the analysed variables of the study are shown in Table 2 as the mean and standard deviation. Regarding the intervention group, a significant decrease in serum concentration was produced for IL-6: patients' anxiety for this group also varied after the diet, significantly decreasing state anxiety, and a significant improvement is shown in functional capacity. Regarding the control group, a significant decrease in the levels of IL-6 in blood is also observed. However, there is no improvement in the level of state or trait anxiety. No change was observed in terms of functional capacity. It is also noteworthy that there was a significant decrease in BMI in both groups.

Table 2. Differences between the study variables after intervention.

IG			
Measure	**Mean**	**SD**	*p*
EDSS pre-test	3.37	2.03	
EDSS post-test	3.28	1.87	0.047 *
IL-6 pre-test (pg/mL)	3.66	4.10	0.000 *
IL-6 post-test (pg/mL)	1.31	2.09	
STAI state pre-test	22.26	8.99	
STAI state post-test	17.67	10.62	0.049 *
STAI trait pre-test	30.11	11.67	
STAI trait post-test	26.89	11.97	0.134
BMI pre-test (kg/m^2)	25.92	5.29	
BMI post-test (kg/m^2)	25.16	4.94	0.002 *
CG			
Measure	**Mean**	**SD**	*p*
EDSS pre-test	3.80	2.00	
EDSS post-test	3.86	2.08	0.655
IL-6 pre-test (pg/mL)	3.67	2.94	0.001 *
IL-6 post-test (pg/mL)	1.37	1.15	
STAI state pre-test	21.71	9.00	
STAI state post-test	21.48	9.39	0.833
STAI trait pre-test	27.04	12.21	
STAI trait post-test	25.83	11.93	0.457
BMI pre-test (kg/m^2)	25.87	6.10	
BMI post-test (kg/m^2)	25.36	5.85	0.012 *

EDSS: Expanded Disability Status Scale; IL-6: interleukin 6 (mean value of normal IL-6, 1.4 pg/mL); STAI: State-Trait Anxiety Inventory; *: statistically significant differences $p < 0.05$; Z: Wilcoxon signed-rank test; BMI: body mass index; SD: standard deviation.

4. Discussion

Among the most representative inflammation biomarkers that activate the immune system caused by stress is IL-6 [36]. This explains that in an immune disease like MS with high oxidative stress, its levels are increased [4]. In this sense, both EGCG and ketone bodies obtained from following ketogenic diets show anti-inflammatory effects [37,38], thus decreasing the levels of IL-6 in blood: EGCG as it negatively regulates its gene expression [39], and ketone bodies block NMDA receptors [40]. After conducting our study, indeed the results prove a decrease in IL-6 levels in the group that received both EGCG and coconut oil. Nonetheless, this significant improvement has also been observed in the control group. This could be explained by the high levels of antioxidants in the Mediterranean diet followed by both groups. The Mediterranean diet is characterised by containing soluble or low molecular weight antioxidants, such as vitamin C and vitamin E, phenolic compounds and carotenoids, and other macromolecular antioxidants that are polymeric phenolic compounds or polyphenols and carotenoids linked to macromolecules of plant foods, which contribute to the antioxidant capacity of the diet [41]; including polyphenols that are greatly contained in fruit and drinks such as tea, red wine and coffee, or in vegetables, pulses and cereals in the Mediterranean diet [30]. In addition, a significant improvement in BMI is observed in both groups that, according to other studies, is positively correlated with IL-6 in blood [42,43], which could explain the decrease in the proinflammatory cytokine in both the control group and the intervention group.

In terms of assessing the psychological variables, although both depression and anxiety disorders are the most frequent nosological entities in MS, the repercussions of symptoms of depression in this pathology have been studied more, and fewer studies assess the impact of anxiety. However, the relation with functional performance and cognitive capacity for MS is only established with levels of anxiety and not with levels of depression [44]. On the other hand, two kinds of anxiety can be differentiated: state anxiety and trait anxiety. According to Spielberger (1972) [45], state anxiety entails an immediate "emotional state" that can be modified in time, while trait anxiety is considered to be relatively stable. In this sense, hyperactivity of the limbic system has been observed in anxiety disorders that could be a result of: a decrease in the inhibitory neurotransmitters (γ-aminobutyric acid, GABA), an increase in the excitatory neurotransmitters based on the action of glutamate or a combination of both [46].

Regarding our intervention, the association of EGCG and ketone bodies causes a significant improvement in state anxiety. This fact seems to be explained through both their action mechanisms. On the one hand, EGCG increases inhibition mediated through the GABA neurotransmitter, which would generate a similar activity to that caused by some medications, such as benzodiazepines [47–49], also decreasing levels of occasional anxiety and causing an anxiolytic effect, as observed after administering it in MS patients [28]. Completing this EGCG activity and based on mechanisms that trigger state anxiety, the action mechanism that ketone bodies have that improves anxiousness [19,20] is based on the inhibition of the activation of NMDA ionotropic glutamate receptors. These receptors have an essential role, not only on a cognitive level [50], but also regarding the presence of anxiety [51]. On the other hand, anxiety is felt both on a physiological level, as well as on a cognitive and a mental level [52]; therefore, symptoms have a negative effect on the cognitive function of those who suffer from anxiety. Anxiety symptoms are especially associated with a lower cognitive function [53] in MS, showing a similar pattern to that observed in people with other immune-mediated inflammatory diseases (IMID) and in individuals without an IMID [54]. Therefore, anxiety in MS patients is related to functional disability and constitutes an indicator of the level of this disability [15]. Our results are in line with this idea, as the patients from the intervention group whose levels of anxiety decrease also show a significant improvement in functional capacity. Nonetheless, we must remember that regarding the two types of anxiety, it is state anxiety that significantly improved, therefore it seems that functionality is more directly related to this kind of anxiety and not trait anxiety. These findings would be supported by the results obtained by other authors, who observed how state anxiety (consisting of a temporary emotional state or condition of the human organism that can vary over time and whose intensity can vary), yet not trait anxiety, predicts the performance in the executive function index. Thus, we can conclude that improving state anxiety improves patients' functionality [44].

However, these results need to be confirmed as this study is somewhat limited. These limitations include a small sample and the lack of intervention groups to study the single contribution of EGCG and coconut oil to improve different variables. Therefore, future research should involve a larger sample leading to a more complex statistical analysis, as well as studying different groups of patients using EGCG, coconut oil and Mediterranean diet, separately.

5. Conclusions

Once the intervention with MS patients was carried out, we observed a decrease in state anxiety, and possibly as a result of this, an improvement in the functional capacity of these patients. However, these improvements do not seem to be a direct consequence of the decrease of IL-6 levels in blood, as this can be observed in both groups (intervention group and control group). This could be due to the antioxidant capacity of the Mediterranean diet that all participants of the study followed, as well as the improvements that this diet shows in terms of BMI.

Author Contributions: Conceptualisation, J.E.d.l.R.O. and J.L.P.; data curation, M.C.-B. and E.D.; formal analysis, J.E.d.l.R.O. and M.M.L.-R.; investigation, M.C.-B., E.D. and J.L.P.; methodology, M.M.L.-R., E.D., V.I. and D.S.; resources, M.C.-B. and D.S.; software, M.M.L.-R.; validation, V.I. and D.S.; writing—original draft, J.E.d.l.R.O.;

writing—review and editing, J.E.d.l.R.O., M.M.L.-R. and J.L.P. All authors have read and agreed to the published version of the manuscript.

Funding: This research was funded by the Catholic University Foundation San Vicente Mártir, for the research project "The Impact of Triglycerides on Multiple Sclerosis" (promotion code 2018-203-001).

Acknowledgments: The authors would like to thank the Health Sciences Research Group CTS-451 from the University of Almería (Spain) for its support. We would also like to thank the MS patients who took part in this study, especially Carmen Farinos.

Conflicts of Interest: The authors declare no conflict of interest.

References

1. McFarland, H.F.; Martin, R. Multiple sclerosis: A complicated picture of autoimmunity. *Nat. Immunol.* **2007**, *8*, 913–919. [CrossRef]

2. Constantinescu, C.S.; Gran, B. Multiple sclerosis: Autoimmune associations in multiple sclerosis. *Nat. Rev. Neurol.* **2010**, *6*, 591. [CrossRef] [PubMed]

3. Kutzelnigg, A.; Lassmann, H. Pathology of multiple sclerosis and related inflammatory demyelinating diseases. *Handb. Clin. Neurol.* **2014**, *122*, 15–58. [CrossRef] [PubMed]

4. Stelmasiak, Z.; Koziol-Montewka, M.; Dobosz, B.; Rejdak, K.; Bartosik-Psujek, H.; Mitosek-Szewczyk, K.; Belniak-Legiec, E. Interleukin-6 concentration in serum and cerebrospinal fluid in multiple sclerosis patients. *Med. Sci. Monit.* **2000**, *6*, 1104–1108. [PubMed]

5. Bongioanni, P.; Mosti, S.; Romano, M.R.; Lombardo, F.; Moscato, G.; Meucci, G. Increased T-lymphocyte interleukin-6 binding in patients with multiple sclerosis. *Eur. J. Neurol.* **2000**, *7*, 291–297. [CrossRef]

6. Goh, V.H.; Tain, C.F.; Tong, T.Y.; Mok, H.P.; Wong, M.T. Are BMI and other anthropometric measures appropriate as indices for obesity? A study in an Asian population. *J. Lipid Res.* **2004**, *45*, 1892–1898. [CrossRef]

7. Kryst, L.; Zeglen, M.; Wronka, I.; Woronkowicz, A.; Bilinska-Pawlak, I.; Das, R.; Saha, R.; Das, S.; Dasgupta, P. Anthropometric variations in different BMI and adiposity levels among children, adolescents and young adults in Kolkata, India. *J. Biosoc. Sci.* **2019**, *51*, 603–618. [CrossRef]

8. Yan, J.; Liu, J.; Lin, C.Y.; Csurhes, P.A.; Pender, M.P.; McCombe, P.A.; Greer, J.M. Interleukin-6 gene promoter-572 C allele may play a role in rate of disease progression in multiple sclerosis. *Int. J. Mol. Sci.* **2012**, *13*, 13667–13679. [CrossRef]

9. Hoge, E.A.; Brandstetter, K.; Moshier, S.; Pollack, M.H.; Wong, K.K.; Simon, N.M. Broad spectrum of cytokine abnormalities in panic disorder and posttraumatic stress disorder. *Depress Anxiety* **2009**, *26*, 447–455. [CrossRef]

10. O'Donovan, A.; Hughes, B.M.; Slavich, G.M.; Lynch, L.; Cronin, M.T.; O'Farrelly, C.; Malone, K.M. Clinical anxiety, cortisol and interleukin-6: Evidence for specificity in emotion-biology relationships. *Brain Behav. Immun.* **2010**, *24*, 1074–1077. [CrossRef]

11. Maes, M.; Song, C.; Lin, A.; De Jongh, R.; Van Gastel, A.; Kenis, G.; Bosmans, E.; De Meester, I.; Benoy, I.; Neels, H.; et al. The effects of psychological stress on humans: Increased production of pro-inflammatory cytokines and a Th1-like response in stress-induced anxiety. *Cytokine* **1998**, *10*, 313–318. [CrossRef] [PubMed]

12. Niraula, A.; Witcher, K.G.; Sheridan, J.F.; Godbout, J.P. Interleukin-6 Induced by Social Stress Promotes a Unique Transcriptional Signature in the Monocytes That Facilitate Anxiety. *Biol. Psychiatry* **2019**, *85*, 679–689. [CrossRef] [PubMed]

13. Malygin, V.L.; Boyko, A.N.; Konovalova, O.E.; Pahtusova, E.E.; Dumbrova, E.V.; Tishina, I.A.; Malygin, Y.V. Anxiety and depressive psychopathological characteristics of patients with multiple sclerosis at different stages of disease. *Zhurnal Nevrologii i Psikhiatrii Imeni SS Korsakova* **2019**, *119*, 58–63. [CrossRef] [PubMed]

14. Genova, H.M.; Lancaster, K.; Lengenfelder, J.; Bober, C.P.; DeLuca, J.; Chiaravalloti, N.D. Relationship between social cognition and fatigue, depressive symptoms, and anxiety in multiple sclerosis. *J. Neuropsychol.* **2019**. [CrossRef] [PubMed]

15. Askari, F.; Ghajarzadeh, M.; Mohammadifar, M.; Azimi, A.; Sahraian, M.A.; Owji, M. Anxiety in patients with multiple sclerosis: Association with disability, depression, disease type and sex. *Acta Med. Iran.* **2014**, *52*, 889–892. [PubMed]

16. Gershuni, V.M.; Yan, S.L.; Medici, V. Nutritional Ketosis for Weight Management and Reversal of Metabolic Syndrome. *Curr. Nutr. Rep.* **2018**, *7*, 97–106. [CrossRef]

17. Offermanns, S.; Schwaninger, M. Nutritional or pharmacological activation of HCA(2) ameliorates neuroinflammation. *Trends Mol. Med.* **2015**, *21*, 245–255. [CrossRef]

18. Rahman, M.; Muhammad, S.; Khan, M.A.; Chen, H.; Ridder, D.A.; Muller-Fielitz, H.; Pokorna, B.; Vollbrandt, T.; Stolting, I.; Nadrowitz, R.; et al. The beta-hydroxybutyrate receptor HCA2 activates a neuroprotective subset of macrophages. *Nat. Commun.* **2014**, *5*, 3944. [CrossRef]

19. Kashiwaya, Y.; Bergman, C.; Lee, J.H.; Wan, R.; King, M.T.; Mughal, M.R.; Okun, E.; Clarke, K.; Mattson, M.P.; Veech, R.L. A ketone ester diet exhibits anxiolytic and cognition-sparing properties, and lessens amyloid and tau pathologies in a mouse model of Alzheimer's disease. *Neurobiol. Aging* **2013**, *34*, 1530–1539. [CrossRef]

20. Fidianingsih, I.; Jamil, N.A.; Andriani, R.N.; Rindra, W.M. Decreased anxiety after Dawood fasting in the pre-elderly and elderly. *J. Complement. Integr. Med.* **2018**, *16*. [CrossRef]

21. Bezard, J.; Bugaut, M.; Clement, G. Triglyceride composition of coconut oil. *J. Am. Oil Chem. Soc.* **1971**, *48*, 134–139. [CrossRef]

22. Pehowich, D.J.; Gomes, A.V.; Barnes, J.A. Fatty acid composition and possible health effects of coconut constituents. *West Indian Med. J.* **2000**, *49*, 128–133. [PubMed]

23. Singh, B.N.; Shankar, S.; Srivastava, R.K. Green tea catechin, epigallocatechin-3-gallate (EGCG): Mechanisms, perspectives and clinical applications. *Biochem. Pharmacol.* **2011**, *82*, 1807–1821. [CrossRef]

24. Riegsecker, S.; Wiczynski, D.; Kaplan, M.J.; Ahmed, S. Potential benefits of green tea polyphenol EGCG in the prevention and treatment of vascular inflammation in rheumatoid arthritis. *Life Sci.* **2013**, *93*, 307–312. [CrossRef]

25. Wu, D.; Wang, J.; Pae, M.; Meydani, S.N. Green tea EGCG, T cells, and T cell-mediated autoimmune diseases. *Mol. Asp. Med.* **2012**, *33*, 107–118. [CrossRef]

26. Lin, L.C.; Wang, M.N.; Tseng, T.Y.; Sung, J.S.; Tsai, T.H. Pharmacokinetics of (-)-epigallocatechin-3-gallate in conscious and freely moving rats and its brain regional distribution. *J. Agric. Food Chem.* **2007**, *55*, 1517–1524. [CrossRef]

27. Schroeder, E.K.; Kelsey, N.A.; Doyle, J.; Breed, E.; Bouchard, R.J.; Loucks, F.A.; Harbison, R.A.; Linseman, D.A. Green tea epigallocatechin 3-gallate accumulates in mitochondria and displays a selective antiapoptotic effect against inducers of mitochondrial oxidative stress in neurons. *Antioxid. Redox Signal.* **2009**, *11*, 469–480. [CrossRef]

28. Johnston, G.A. Flavonoid nutraceuticals and ionotropic receptors for the inhibitory neurotransmitter GABA. *Neurochem. Int.* **2015**, *89*, 120–125. [CrossRef]

29. Loftis, J.M.; Wilhelm, C.J.; Huckans, M. Effect of epigallocatechin gallate supplementation in schizophrenia and bipolar disorder: An 8-week, randomized, double-blind, placebo-controlled study. *Ther. Adv. Psychopharmacol.* **2013**, *3*, 21–27. [CrossRef]

30. Manach, C.; Scalbert, A.; Morand, C.; Remesy, C.; Jimenez, L. Polyphenols: Food sources and bioavailability. *Am. J. Clin. Nutr.* **2004**, *79*, 727–747. [CrossRef]

31. Spielberger, C.D. State-Trait anxiety inventory. In *The Corsini Encyclopedia of Psychology*; Wiley Online Library: Hoboken, NJ, USA, 2010.

32. Spielberger, C.D.; Díaz-Guerrero, R. *Idare: Inventario de Ansiedad: Rasgo-Estado*; Editorial El Manual Moderno: Mexico City, Mexico, 1975.

33. Rojas-Carrasco, K.E. Validación del Inventario de Ansiedad Rasgo-Estado en padres con un hijo en terapia intensiva. *Rev. Med. Inst. Mex. Seguro Soc.* **2010**, *48*, 491–496.

34. Kurtzke, J.F. Rating neurologic impairment in multiple sclerosis: An expanded disability status scale (EDSS). *Neurology* **1983**, *33*, 1444–1452. [CrossRef] [PubMed]

35. World Medical, A. World Medical Association Declaration of Helsinki: Ethical principles for medical research involving human subjects. *JAMA* **2013**, *310*, 2191–2194. [CrossRef]

36. Morera, L.P.; Tempesti, T.C.; Pérez, E.; Medrano, L.A. Biomarcadores en la medición del estrés: Una revisión sistemática. *Ansiedad y Estrés* **2019**, *25*, 49–58. [CrossRef]

37. Shan, L.; Kang, X.; Liu, F.; Cai, X.; Han, X.; Shang, Y. Epigallocatechin gallate improves airway inflammation through TGFbeta1 signaling pathway in asthmatic mice. *Mol. Med. Rep.* **2018**, *18*, 2088–2096. [CrossRef] [PubMed]

38. Anez-Bustillos, L.; Dao, D.T.; Finkelstein, A.; Pan, A.; Cho, B.S.; Mitchell, P.D.; Gura, K.M.; Bistrian, B.R.; Puder, M. Metabolic and Inflammatory Effects of an omega-3 Fatty Acid-Based Eucaloric Ketogenic Diet in Mice With Endotoxemia. *JPEN* **2019**, *43*, 986–997. [CrossRef] [PubMed]

39. Huang, H.Y.; Wang, M.C.; Chen, Z.Y.; Chiu, W.Y.; Chen, K.H.; Lin, I.C.; Yang, W.V.; Wu, C.C.; Tseng, C.L. Gelatin-epigallocatechin gallate nanoparticles with hyaluronic acid decoration as eye drops can treat rabbit dry-eye syndrome effectively via inflammatory relief. *Int. J. Nanomed.* **2018**, *13*, 7251–7273. [CrossRef]

40. Amani, M.; Zolghadrnasab, M.; Salari, A.A. NMDA receptor in the hippocampus alters neurobehavioral phenotypes through inflammatory cytokines in rats with sporadic Alzheimer-like disease. *Physiol. Behav.* **2019**, *202*, 52–61. [CrossRef]

41. Perez-Jimenez, J.; Diaz-Rubio, M.E.; Saura-Calixto, F. Contribution of Macromolecular Antioxidants to Dietary Antioxidant Capacity: A Study in the Spanish Mediterranean Diet. *Plant Foods Hum. Nutr.* **2015**, *70*, 365–370. [CrossRef]

42. De Filippo, G.; Rendina, D.; Moccia, F.; Rocco, V.; Campanozzi, A. Interleukin-6, soluble interleukin-6 receptor/interleukin-6 complex and insulin resistance in obese children and adolescents. *J. Endocrinol. Investig.* **2015**, *38*, 339–343. [CrossRef]

43. Tucker, P.; Pfefferbaum, B.; Nitiema, P.; Khan, Q.; Aggarwal, R.; Walling, E.E. Possible link of Interleukin-6 and Interleukin-2 with psychiatric diagnosis, ethnicity, disaster or BMI. *Cytokine* **2017**, *96*, 247–252. [CrossRef] [PubMed]

44. Julian, L.J.; Arnett, P.A. Relationships among anxiety, depression, and executive functioning in multiple sclerosis. *Clin. Neuropsychol.* **2009**, *23*, 794–804. [CrossRef] [PubMed]

45. Spielberger, C.D. *Anxiety: Current Trends in Theory and Research*; Elsevier: Amsterdam, The Netherlands, 2013; pp. 23–49.

46. Martin, E.I.; Ressler, K.J.; Binder, E.; Nemeroff, C.B. The neurobiology of anxiety disorders: Brain imaging, genetics, and psychoneuroendocrinology. *Psychiatr. Clin. N. Am.* **2009**, *32*, 549–575. [CrossRef] [PubMed]

47. Vignes, M.; Maurice, T.; Lante, F.; Nedjar, M.; Thethi, K.; Guiramand, J.; Recasens, M. Anxiolytic properties of green tea polyphenol (-)-epigallocatechin gallate (EGCG). *Brain Res.* **2006**, *1110*, 102–115. [CrossRef] [PubMed]

48. Lee, B.; Shim, I.; Lee, H.; Hahm, D.H. Effects of Epigallocatechin Gallate on Behavioral and Cognitive Impairments, Hypothalamic-Pituitary-Adrenal Axis Dysfunction, and Alternations in Hippocampal BDNF Expression under Single Prolonged Stress. *J. Med. Food* **2018**, *21*, 979–989. [CrossRef]

49. Camfield, D.A.; Stough, C.; Farrimond, J.; Scholey, A.B. Acute effects of tea constituents L-theanine, caffeine, and epigallocatechin gallate on cognitive function and mood: A systematic review and meta-analysis. *Nutr. Rev.* **2014**, *72*, 507–522. [CrossRef]

50. Castellano, C.; Cestari, V.; Ciamei, A. NMDA receptors and learning and memory processes. *Curr. Drug Targets* **2001**, *2*, 273–283. [CrossRef]

51. Barkus, C.; McHugh, S.B.; Sprengel, R.; Seeburg, P.H.; Rawlins, J.N.; Bannerman, D.M. Hippocampal NMDA receptors and anxiety: At the interface between cognition and emotion. *Eur. J. Pharmacol.* **2010**, *626*, 49–56. [CrossRef]

52. Fernandez-Rodriguez, M.; Rodriguez-Legorburu, I.; Lopez-Ibor Alcocer, M.I. Nutritional supplements in Anxiety Disorder. *Actas Esp. Psiquiatr.* **2017**, *45*, 1–7.

53. Oreja-Guevara, C.; Ayuso Blanco, T.; Brieva Ruiz, L.; Hernandez Perez, M.A.; Meca-Lallana, V.; Ramio-Torrenta, L. Cognitive Dysfunctions and Assessments in Multiple Sclerosis. *Front. Neurol.* **2019**, *10*, 581. [CrossRef]

54. Whitehouse, C.E.; Fisk, J.D.; Bernstein, C.N.; Berrigan, L.I.; Bolton, J.M.; Graff, L.A.; Hitchon, C.A.; Marriott, J.J.; Peschken, C.A.; Sareen, J.; et al. Comorbid anxiety, depression, and cognition in MS and other immune-mediated disorders. *Neurology* **2019**. [CrossRef] [PubMed]

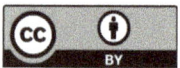

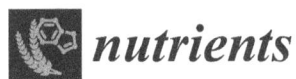

Article

Association between Depressive Symptoms and Food Insecurity among Indonesian Adults: Results from the 2007–2014 Indonesia Family Life Survey

Emyr Reisha Isaura [1,2], **Yang-Ching Chen** [2,3,4], **Annis Catur Adi** [1,5], **Hsien-Yu Fan** [4], **Chung-Yi Li** [1,6] and **Shwu-Huey Yang** [2,7,8,*]

[1] Department of Nutrition, Faculty of Public Health, Airlangga University, Surabaya, East Java 60115, Indonesia; emyr.reisha@fkm.unair.ac.id (E.R.I.); annis_catur@fkm.unair.ac.id (A.C.A.); cyli99@mail.ncku.edu.tw (C.-Y.L.)

[2] School of Nutrition and Health Sciences, College of Nutrition, Taipei Medical University, Taipei 11031, Taiwan; melisa26@gmail.com

[3] Department of Family Medicine, School of Medicine, College of Medicine, Taipei Medical University, Taipei 11031, Taiwan

[4] Department of Family Medicine, Taipei Medical University Hospital, Taipei 11031, Taiwan; a1118148@ulive.pccu.edu.tw

[5] Research Center of Food Science and Technology, Rumah Inovasi Natura, Surabaya, East Java 60112, Indonesia

[6] Department and Graduate Institute of Public Health, College of Medicine, National Cheng Kung University, Tainan 70101, Taiwan

[7] Nutrition Research Center, Taipei Medical University Hospital, Taipei 11031, Taiwan

[8] Research Center of Geriatric Nutrition, College of Nutrition, Taipei Medical University, Taipei 11031, Taiwan

* Correspondence: sherry@tmu.edu.tw; Tel.: +886-2-2736-1661 (ext. 6568)

Received: 5 November 2019; Accepted: 10 December 2019; Published: 11 December 2019

Abstract: Background: Depressive symptoms and food insecurity are two of the public health concerns in developing countries. Food insecurity is linked to several chronic diseases, while little is known about the association between food insecurity and depressive symptoms among adults. A person with limited or uncertain availability or access to nutritionally sufficient, socially relevant, and safe foods is defined as a food-insecure person. Materials and methods: Data were obtained from 8613 adults who participated in the Indonesia Family Life Survey (IFLS) in 2007 and 2014. The 10 items of the food frequency questionnaire (FFQ) were used in food consumption score analysis to assess food insecurity based on the concept of the World Food Program (WFP). Depressive symptoms were assessed using 10 items of the self-reported Center for Epidemiologic Studies Depression (CES-D) questionnaire. A linear and multiple logistic regression model with a generalized estimating equation was used to test the hypothesis while accounting for the health behaviors and sociodemographic characteristics. Results: Food consumption score was negatively associated with CES-D 10 score (β-coefficients: -9.71×10^{-3} to -1.06×10^{-2}; 95% CIs: -7.46×10^{-3} to -1.26×10^{-2}). The borderline and poor food consumption group was positively associated with the depressive symptoms, both in the unadjusted and adjusted models (exponentiated β-coefficients: 1.13 to 1.18; 95% CIs: 1.06 to 1.28). Conclusions: Depressive symptoms were positively significantly associated with food insecurity. Thus, health professionals must be aware of the issue, and should consider health and nutrition programs for adults at risk of food insecurity.

Keywords: depressive symptoms; food insecurity; nutrition; adults; generalized estimating equation

1. Introduction

Depression is a public health problem, associated with adverse mental health, such as suicidal ideation and mortality [1]. Depression is defined as a wide range of mental health problems associated with the negative effect presence, low mood, and emotional, cognitive, physical, and behavioral symptoms [2]. Depression is also a pervasive mental disorder globally that affects all ages [3]. In 2012, depression was estimated to affect about 350 million people globally [3]. Further, the global population with depression was estimated to be 4.4% in 2015, while Indonesia's national prevalence rate for people having depressive symptoms is 3.7% [4]. Depression or depressive symptoms can occur in episodic sequences [2]. Some unwanted life events (e.g., the loss of a loved one or separation in a relationship), or living with poverty, being unemployed, having a physical illness, and drug and alcohol use-related problems, increase the risk of depression or having depressive symptoms [4,5]. Furthermore, an adult who is unemployed or living in poverty is also associated with food insecurity because of the financial resource limits for acquiring food and managing their diet [6].

Food insecurity is defined as a condition in which a person has limited or uncertain availability or access to nutritionally adequate, culturally relevant, and safe foods [6]. Moreover, food insecurity has been found to be associated with chronic diseases [7,8]. The former researchers suggested that chronic diseases may be a contributing factor in the association between food insecurity and depression among the elderly [9–11]. On the other hand, food-insecure people are prone to consume an energy-dense and less diverse diet, which eventually results in overweight and obesity, and a higher risk of hypertension, diabetes, and cardiovascular diseases [7,8,12,13]. Seligman and Schillinger suggested that there is a trade-off between providing food and buying medicine in the association between food insecurity, chronic diseases, and depressive symptoms [12]. Not only is the association between food insecurity and depression or depressive symptoms rather vague among adults, but both food insecurity and depression or depressive symptoms can also affect people, women in particular, who live in high-income or low–middle-income countries [14]. Some previous studies found that older adults are prone to the food insecurity issue [15–17]. However, the previous study reported that adults in their forties were faced the severe food insecurity issues [18]. Therefore, in this study we used different methods and study designs to further explore and evaluate whether specific age groups modified the association between food insecurity and depressive symptoms among Indonesian adults. We used repeated measurement data to assess the association between food insecurity and depressive symptoms in adults, both in all ages and in various age groups. In addition, we observed depression or depressive symptoms as both predictor and outcome, and used different food insecurity assessments.

2. Materials and Methods

2.1. Data Source and Respondents

The current study used secondary data from the fourth (2007) and fifth (2014) waves of the Indonesian Family Life Survey (IFLS; referred to hereafter as IFLS4 and IFLS5, respectively). IFLS datasets comprise anonymous data available to researchers based on the guidelines of the RAND Corporation [19–23]. In the 2007 data, the total number of respondents was 29,059, while in 2014, there were 34,464 respondents (aged 0–80+). For this study, we included adult respondents aged 18–65 years old. We included the same respondents from the year 2007 and the year 2014. Respondents who provided dietary, physical activity, anthropometric, sociodemographic, blood pressure, and depressive symptom data were further analyzed. We excluded respondents who were pregnant or breastfeeding, had a disability, or who were diagnosed with cancer to minimize the sampling bias. Further, we included only respondents who had no missing data in both 2007 and 2014. After the inclusion criteria were applied, 8613 respondents were included in this study. For the purposes of this study, the authors additionally categorized respondents' ages in years, as follows: less than 40, 40–49, 50–59, and more than 60, besides using responses as continuous data.

2.2. Measurement of Food Insecurity

Measurement of food insecurity in this study followed the concept from the World Food Program (WFP). In practical terms, the definition of food security is related to the failure of the individual to fulfill their need for a nutritious diet [24] in terms of the frequency and diversity of food [25]. Based on the WFP concept, first, we conducted food consumption analysis, resulting in food consumption scores [26–28]. We used the same 10 types of food from the food frequency questionnaire (FFQ) in the IFLS4 and IFLS5 questionnaire for the food consumption analysis. The current study used the number of days in which the 10 food types were eaten by respondents in the seven days prior to the interview [25]. Second, the 10 food types of the IFLS4 and IFLS5 FFQ were then grouped into five food groups. The five food groups were the vegetable group (carrot, green leafy vegetables), fruit group (mango, papaya, banana), protein group (eggs, fish, meat), dairy products, and staple group (sweet potato) [19,21]. Third, a total from each food group, called the food consumption score (FCS), was then categorized based on the cutoffs of three food consumption groups (FCGs). The FCS is continuous data, while the FCG is categorical data from the categorization of the FCS. The three FCGs were "poor" if the FCS value was less than 21, "borderline" if the FCS value ranged from 21 to 35, and "acceptable" if the value was more than 35 [25]. Finally, this study defined food-insecure people as those who were in the "poor and borderline" group of FCGs, while food-secure people were defined as those in the "acceptable" group of FCG [28,29].

2.3. Measurement of Depressive Symptoms

Depressive symptoms were assessed using the self-reported 10 items of the Center for Epidemiologic Studies Depression (CES-D) questionnaire. The CES-D questionnaire is widely used to assess depressive symptoms in adults [30,31]. The 10 CES-D questionnaire answers were in the form of four scales: "rarely or no ($\leq$1 day)", "some days (1–2 days)", "occasionally (3–4 days)", "most of the time (5–7 days)". The score of each scale's answer was from zero ("rarely or no") to four ("most of the time"). We then summarized the score of the 10 CES-D questionnaire answers with a lowest score of 10, and a highest score of 40. Since the score ranged from 10 to 40, the score was rebased to zero to 30, with the highest score referring to the most depressive symptomatology [30]. Previous research suggested the cutoff point for depression or having depressive symptoms was set to a score of $\geq$10 [30,32,33]. Therefore, respondents were defined as suffering from depression or having depressive symptoms if their CES-D questionnaire score was $\geq$10.

2.4. Measurement of Covariates

The body mass index (in kg/m^2) was classified into four groups (<18.5, 18.5–25.0, 25.1–27.0, and >27.0) [34]. In addition, a measurement of waist circumference was used for adults aged $\geq$40 years. Abdominal obesity was determined by respondents' waist circumference (WC), >90 cm (men) and >80 cm (women) [35]. Hypertension was defined as systolic blood pressure (SBP) $\geq$140 mmHg or diastolic blood pressure (DBP) $\geq$90 mmHg [36]. Trained nurses performed the anthropometric and blood pressure measurements. For blood pressure measurements, the respondents were measured twice, before and during the interview, in the seated position [19].

Physical activity was assessed using the number of days for which respondents undertook three types of physical activity (i.e., vigorous, moderate, and walking) within the last seven days. The authors considered days of doing physical activity as a continuous variable in the analysis. Respondents reported in the self-reported questionnaires whether they engaged in physical activities for at least ten minutes continuously during the last seven days. If respondents said yes, then they were further asked about the number of days they did each type of physical activity.

Sociodemographic characteristics were assessed using categorical data, including smoking habit status, level of education, geographical areas of living, and marital status. The respondents' smoking habit status was categorized into: never (never had a smoking habit), current smoker (currently has a smoking habit), and former smoker (stopped a smoking habit). The respondents' level of education was categorized into low (<12 years of school attainment) and high (≥12 years of school attainment).

In addition to the covariate variables, we considered adjusting for respondents' chronic diseases. Therefore, this study used cardiovascular diseases and type 2 diabetes as an adjustment variable in the model. Respondents answered the self-reported question of whether any paramedics ever informed them that they had type 2 diabetes. The respondents also answered the self-reported question of whether any paramedics ever informed them that they had a stroke/heart attack, coronary heart disease, angina, or other heart problems. The authors defined cardiovascular disease as a combination of heart diseases and stroke events [27,37]. If the respondents reported any of the chronic diseases (i.e., diabetes, cardiovascular diseases), then they were asked when their chronic disease was first diagnosed.

2.5. Statistical Analysis

The current study used secondary data with repeated measurements of the same respondents for the years 2007 and 2014. The respondents' characteristics were presented as means (standard deviation) for the continuous data and numbers (percentages) for the categorical data. The values between groups were compared using a one-way analysis of variance (ANOVA) for the continuous data, and the Bonferroni post-hoc test or chi-squared test for the categorical data. Further, we combined the two datasets (IFLS4 and IFLS5) in the analysis to test the association among variables. Since the data in this study were repeated measurement data from the same respondents throughout the 7-year follow-up period, the authors used regression models with the generalized estimating equation (GEE) method [38]. The GEE is a statistical approach generally used in the analysis of longitudinal data or repeated measurements [39–44], with the primary advantage being that it accounts for the within-adults variation [45]. Firstly, we used a linear regression model with GEE to assess the association between the food consumption score and the CES-D score. The linear regression used the Gaussian distribution (family) for the dependent variables, an identity link function, and "independent" for the correlation matrix. Secondly, we used a binary logistic regression model with GEE to assess the association between food consumption groups and depressive symptoms. The authors used the "acceptable" FCG group as the reference group in the logistic regression model with GEE. The logistic regression model used the "binomial" distribution (family) for the dependent variable, a log link function, and an "independent" correlation matrix. The exponentiated beta coefficient was also estimated from the logistic regression to assess the relationship of interest [45,46]. This study used three models that accounted for various potential confounders in the multiple logistic regression model with GEE. The first model was an unadjusted model and the second model was with an adjustment for age and gender. The third model was with further adjustment for level of education, marital status, geographical areas of living, smoking habit status, physical activity days, blood pressure values, body mass index, and included diabetes and cardiovascular diseases. The last model (model 3) was a full adjustment model. A similar sequence of adjustments for potential confounders was also used for multiple linear regression models with GEE. Statistical significance was set to the p-value < 0.05. The post hoc test was conducted to retest the complete adjustment estimation models for every age group category. All the analyses were conducted using STATA statistical software (V 12.1; StataCorp LP, College Station, Texas, TX, USA).

3. Results

Table 1 shows the characteristics of the 8613 respondents by food security groups in 2007 and 2014. Respondents included 3999 women and 4614 men. The prevalence rates of food insecurity (borderline and poor) increased from 2007 to 2014. The borderline FCG prevalence rates increased from $n = 1474$ (17.11%) in 2007 to $n = 2911$ (33.80%) in 2014. Meanwhile, the prevalence rates of poor FCG also increased from $n = 693$ (8.05%) in 2007 to $n = 1713$ (19.89%) in 2014. The majority of respondents in this study had a low level of education (less than 12 years of school attainment) in both year 2007 and 2014 ($p < 0.001$). The percentage of food-insecure people living in urban areas increased from 2007 (borderline = 18.87%; poor = 9.55%) to 2014 (borderline = 35.31%; poor = 23.46%)

($p < 0.001$). The percentage of food-insecure people with abdominal obesity increased from 2007 (borderline = 15.74%; poor = 6.81%) to 2014 (borderline = 32.75%; poor = 18.00%) ($p < 0.001$). As shown in Table 1, the number of respondents who had depressive symptoms increased from $n = 955$ in 2007 to $n = 2616$ people in 2014. To compare body mass index (BMI), body shape index, waist circumference, blood pressure, food consumption score, physical activity days, and CES-D score, we used a one-way analysis of variance (ANOVA) with Bonferroni post hoc test. The results of the Bonferroni post hoc test are in Tables S1 and S2 of the Supplementary Materials.

Table 2 presents the overall and age-specific proportions of food consumption groups among people with depressive symptoms. In 2007, the overall (range of age-specific proportion) proportion of acceptable, borderline, and poor FCG was 11.65% (range: 0.13%–52.46%), 9.02% (range: 0.75%–54.89%), and 10.24% (range: 0.00%–57.75%), respectively. In 2014, corresponding figures were 32.09% (range: 10.70%–35.70%), 29.34% (range: 10.66%–33.49%), and 28.14% (range: 10.79%–39.63%), respectively. The prevalence of depressive symptoms significantly varied with age. Except for the borderline group in 2007, the proportion of other food consumption groups in both years also significantly varied.

Table 3 demonstrates the association between food consumption groups and the depressive symptoms outcomes among adults. The food consumption score was negatively significantly associated with the CES-D score both in the unadjusted model (β-Coefficients: -9.51×10^{-3} (95% CI: -6.45×10^{-3}, -1.26×10^{-2})) and adjusted models (β-Coefficients: -9.71×10^{-3} (95% CI: -6.62×10^{-3}, -1.28×10^{-2})) to β-Coefficients: -1.04×10^{-2} (95% CI: -7.26×10^{-3}, -1.36×10^{-2})). Further, we used the logistic models to compare food security as represented by acceptable FCG and food insecurity as represented by borderline and poor FCG. The borderline group was positively associated with the depressive symptoms of both the unadjusted and adjusted models with exponentiated β-Coefficients of 1.13 (95% CI: 1.06 to 1.21) to 1.18 (95% CI: 1.10 to 1.26). The depressive symptoms of the borderline group will increase by 1.13–1.18 units for every one-unit increase of the acceptable group. On the other hand, the poor group was also significantly positively associated with the depressive symptoms in both the unadjusted and adjusted models, with exponentiated β-Coefficients of 1.17 (95% CI: 1.07 to 1.27) to 1.22 (95% CI: 1.12 to 1.33). The depressive symptoms of the poor group will increase by 1.17–1.22 units for every one-unit increase of the acceptable group.

Table 4 shows the results of age-specific analyses for the relationship between food insecurity (as represented by FCS and FGC) and depression or depressive symptoms (as represented by the CES-D score). The current study used a full adjustment model (model 3) in the analysis to examine the findings' post hoc stability and decide whether the regression analysis differed based on the age group. The poor food consumption group was significantly and independently positively associated with depressive symptoms among respondents aged 40–49 years, with an exponentiated β-Coefficient of 1.24 (95% CI: 1.08 to 1.42). The depressive symptoms of the poor food consumption group will increase by 1.24 units for every one-unit increase of the acceptable food consumption group only among respondents aged 40–49 years. The remaining age groups did not report a food consumption score nor food consumption groups that were significantly associated with depressive symptoms.

Table 1. Respondents' characteristics by food security group.

	2007				2014			
	Acceptable	Borderline	Poor	p-Value	Acceptable	Borderline	Poor	p-Value
n (%)	6446 (74.84)	1474 (17.11)	693 (8.05)		3989 (46.31)	2911 (33.80)	1713 (19.89)	
Age (years), mean (SD)	41 (9)	40 (9)	41 (9)	0.110	48 (9)	47 (9)	48 (9)	0.004
Age (years), n (%)								
<40	2946 (74.64)	705 (17.86)	296 (7.50)		918 (45.22)	743 (36.60)	369 (18.18)	
40–59	2210 (75.81)	472 (16.19)	233 (7.99)		1357 (47.58)	949 (33.27)	546 (19.14)	
50–59	1286 (73.70)	295 (16.91)	164 (9.40)		1243 (46.42)	881 (32.90)	554 (20.69)	
≥60	4 (66.67)	2 (33.33)	0 (0.00)		471 (44.73)	338 (32.10)	244 (23.17)	
Sex, n (%)				0.021				0.034
Women	2937 (73.44)	721 (18.03)	341 (8.53)		1799 (44.99)	1365 (34.13)	835 (20.88)	
Men	3509 (76.05)	753 (16.32)	352 (7.63)		2190 (47.46)	1546 (33.51)	878 (19.03)	
Level of Education, n (%)				<0.001				<0.001
Low (<12 years attainment)	4162 (70.00)	1185 (19.93)	599 (10.07)		2365 (40.27)	2054 (34.97)	1454 (24.76)	
High (≥12 years attainment)	2284 (85.64)	289 (10.84)	94 (3.52)		1624 (59.27)	857 (31.28)	259 (9.45)	
Marital Status, n (%)				0.231				0.309
Married or ever married	5954 (74.76)	1358 (17.05)	652 (8.19)		3854 (46.33)	2820 (33.90)	1645 (19.77)	
Single or Never Married	492 (75.81)	116 (17.87)	41 (6.32)		135 (45.92)	91 (30.95)	68 (23.13)	
Geographical areas of living, n (%)				<0.001				<0.001
Rural	3050 (71.58)	804 (18.87)	407 (9.55)		1471 (41.23)	1260 (35.31)	837 (23.46)	
Urban	3396 (78.03)	670 (15.40)	286 (6.57)		2518 (49.91)	1651 (32.73)	876 (17.36)	
Smoking Habit Status, n (%)				0.124				0.003
Never	3827 (75.22)	864 (16.98)	397 (7.80)		2271 (46.61)	1639 (33.64)	962 (19.75)	
Current Smoker	2461 (73.90)	582 (17.48)	287 (8.62)		1440 (44.65)	1116 (34.60)	669 (20.74)	
Former smoker	158 (81.03)	28 (14.36)	9 (4.62)		278 (53.88)	156 (30.23)	82 (15.89)	
Using Diabetes Medication, n (%)				0.622				0.468
No	6437 (74.85)	1472 (17.12)	691 (8.03)		3925 (46.24)	2872 (33.83)	1692 (19.93)	
Yes	9 (69.23)	2 (15.38)	2 (15.38)		64 (51.61)	39 (31.45)	21 (16.94)	
Using Hypertension Medication, n (%)				0.173				0.007
No	6391 (74.77)	1468 (17.17)	689 (8.06)		3796 (46.01)	2794 (33.86)	1661 (20.13)	
Yes	55 (84.62)	6 (9.23)	4 (6.15)		193 (53.31)	117 (32.32)	52 (14.36)	
Using Cholesterol Medication, n (%)				0.557				0.002
No	6442 (74.85)	1472 (17.10)	692 (8.04)		3906 (46.08)	2876 (33.93)	1695 (20.00)	
Yes	4 (57.14)	2 (28.57)	1 (14.29)		83 (61.03)	35 (25.74)	18 (13.24)	

Table 1. *Cont.*

	2007				2014			
	Acceptable	Borderline	Poor	p-Value	Acceptable	Borderline	Poor	p-Value
Abdominal obesity †, n (%)				0.001				<0.001
No	2108 (73.48)	485 (16.90)	276 (9.62)		1556 (44.43)	1158 (33.07)	788 (22.50)	
Yes	1388 (77.46)	282 (15.74)	122 (6.81)		1516 (49.25)	1008 (32.75)	554 (18.00)	
Body Mass Index (kg/m²), mean (SD)	23.31 (4.16)	22.86 (4.09)	22.50 (4.07)	<0.001	24.31 (4.33)	24.10 (4.44)	23.42 (4.31)	<0.001
Body Mass Index ‡, n (%)				<0.001				<0.001
<18.5	562 (70.07)	154 (19.20)	86 (10.72)		285 (41.07)	242 (34.87)	167 (24.06)	
18.5–25.0	3978 (74.02)	943 (17.55)	453 (8.43)		2099 (44.74)	1570 (33.46)	1023 (21.80)	
25.1–27.0	771 (78.19)	147 (14.91)	68 (6.90)		610 (50.12)	412 (33.85)	195 (16.02)	
>27.0	1135 (78.22)	230 (15.85)	86 (5.93)		995 (49.50)	687 (34.18)	328 (16.32)	
Hypertension, n (%)				0.716				0.093
No	4485 (75.09)	1014 (16.98)	474 (7.94)		2410 (46.59)	1773 (34.27)	990 (19.14)	
Yes	1961 (74.28)	460 (17.42)	219 (8.30)		1579 (45.90)	1138 (33.08)	723 (21.02)	
Diabetes, n (%)				0.182				0.660
No	6431 (74.88)	1468 (17.09)	689 (8.02)		3854 (46.24)	2817 (33.80)	1663 (19.95)	
Yes	15 (60.0)	6 (24.00)	4 (16.00)		135 (48.39)	94 (33.69)	50 (17.92)	
Cardiovascular Disease, n (%)				0.097				0.424
No	6390 (74.75)	1467 (17.16)	691 (8.08)		3886 (46.32)	2828 (33.71)	1675 (19.97)	
Yes	56 (86.15)	7 (10.77)	2 (3.08)		103 (45.98)	83 (37.05)	38 (16.96)	
Depression *, n (%)				0.011				0.004
No	5695 (74.37)	1341 (17.51)	622 (8.12)		2709 (45.17)	2057 (34.30)	1231 (20.53)	
Yes	751 (78.64)	133 (13.93)	71 (7.43)		1280 (48.93)	854 (32.65)	482 (18.43)	
Body Shape Index (m$^{11/6}$ kg$^{-2/3}$), mean (SD)	0.0814 (0.0056)	0.0816 (0.0059)	0.0815 (0.0056)	0.028	0.0814 (0.0056)	0.0815 (0.0056)	0.0816 (0.0059)	0.726
Waist Circumference (cm), mean (SD)	82.22 (10.86)	80.70 (10.62)	79.10 (10.77)	<0.001	85.29 (11.51)	84.47 (11.50)	82.70 (12.00)	<0.001
Systolic BP (mmHg), mean (SD)	129.72 (19.12)	130.43 (19.82)	130.86 (19.52)	0.184	135.51 (23.07)	136.31 (23.88)	138.09 (23.72)	<0.001
Diastolic BP (mmHg), mean (SD)	81.41 (11.64)	81.49 (11.48)	81.25 (10.65)	0.899	82.93 (13.16)	83.22 (13.33)	83.35 (13.27)	0.467
Food Consumption Score, mean (SD)	60.71 (18.26)	29.32 (3.90)	15.07 (4.90)	<0.001	46.99 (10.68)	29.81 (4.04)	13.69 (5.43)	<0.001
Walking PA Days, mean (SD)	4 (3)	4 (3)	4 (3)	0.264	4 (3)	4 (3)	4 (3)	0.149
Moderate PA Days, mean (SD)	3 (3)	2 (3)	2 (3)	0.001	3 (3)	2 (3)	2 (3)	0.001
Vigorous PA Days, mean (SD)	1 (2)	1 (2)	1 (2)	0.207	1 (2)	1 (2)	1 (2)	0.019
CES-D 10 Score, mean (SD)	6.19 (3.29)	5.77 (3.16)	5.48 (3.58)	<0.001	8.37 (4.81)	7.93 (4.90)	7.59 (5.24)	<0.001

Notes: BP, blood pressures; PA, physical activity; CES-D 10, Center for Epidemiological Studies Depression 10 items; SD, standard deviation. n (%) was for categorical data and mean (SD) was for continuous data presentation. † A definition of abdominal obesity was if women had waist circumference >80 cm or men had waist circumference >90 cm. ‡ Body Mass Index used the cutoff values for the Indonesian adults from the Ministry of Health of Indonesia. * Depression = CES-D 10 score ≥10.

43

Table 2. The food consumption groups co-occurring with depressive symptoms by age among adults.

	All ages	<40	40-59	50-59	≥60	p-Value
2007						
Depressive Symptoms, *n* (%)	955 (11.09)	508 (53.19)	294 (30.79)	151 (15.81)	2 (0.21)	<0.001
Food Consumption Groups, *n* (%)						
Acceptable	751 (11.65)	394 (52.46)	235 (31.29)	121 (16.11)	1 (0.13)	0.001
Borderline	133 (9.02)	73 (54.89)	38 (28.57)	21 (15.79)	1 (0.75)	0.059
Poor	71 (10.24)	41 (57.75)	21 (29.58)	9 (12.68)	0 (0.0)	0.014
2014						
Depressive Symptoms, *n* (%)	2616 (30.4)	719 (27.48)	934 (35.70)	683 (26.11)	280 (10.70)	<0.001
Food Consumption Groups, *n* (%)						
Acceptable	1280 (32.09)	349 (27.27)	457 (35.70)	337 (26.33)	137 (10.70)	<0.001
Borderline	854 (29.34)	251 (29.39)	286 (33.49)	226 (26.46)	91 (10.66)	0.003
Poor	482 (28.14)	119 (24.69)	191 (39.63)	120 (24.90)	52 (10.79)	<0.001

Notes: Depressive symptoms were defined as CES-D 10 score ≥10. Prevalence rates are shown as numbers (weighted prevalence). Depression rates between food consumption groups within the age group were significant (p-value = 0.004–0.011).

Table 3. The association between food consumption groups and the depressive symptoms outcomes among adults.

Variables	Model 1		Model 2		Model 3	
	β (95% CI)	p-Value	β (95% CI)	p-Value	β (95% CI)	p-Value
FCS	-9.51×10^{-3} $(-6.45 \times 10^{-3}, -1.26 \times 10^{-2})$	<0.001	-9.71×10^{-3} $(-6.62 \times 10^{-3}, -1.28 \times 10^{-2})$	<0.001	-1.06×10^{-2} $(-7.46 \times 10^{-3}, -1.38 \times 10^{-2})$	<0.001
Acceptable	1 (Ref.)		1 (Ref.)		1 (Ref.)	
Borderline*	1.16 (1.08–1.24)	<0.001	1.15 (1.08–1.23)	<0.001	1.13 (1.06–1.21)	<0.001
Poor*	1.18 (1.09–1.28)	<0.001	1.17 (1.08–1.27)	<0.001	1.17 (1.07–1.27)	<0.001

Notes: CI, confidence interval; FCS, food consumption score. FCS is continuous data of the food security assessment. Depressive symptoms were defined as CES-D 10 score ≥10. Model 1: Unadjusted model. Model 2: Model 1 with adjustment for age and gender. Model 2 with adjustment for level of education, marital status, geographical areas of living, smoking habit status, physical activity days, blood pressures, body mass index, diabetes, and cardiovascular diseases. * The exponentiated β-coefficient was used for the logistic models of generalized estimating equation.

Table 4. The association between food consumption groups and the depressive symptoms outcomes among adults by specific age group.

Variables	<40 years		40–49 years		50–59 years		≥60 years	
	β (95% CI)	*p*-value	β (95% CI)	*p*-Value	β (95% CI)	*p*-Value	β (95% CI)	*p*-Value
FCS	1.65×10^{-3} $(-5.43 \times 10^{-3}, 8.73 \times 10^{-3})$	0.649	-4.27×10^{-3} $(-9.99 \times 10^{-3}, 1.46 \times 10^{-3})$	0.144	1.11×10^{-3} $(-4.47 \times 10^{-3}, 6.70 \times 10^{-3})$	0.696	5.43×10^{-3} $(-3.63 \times 10^{-3}, 1.45 \times 10^{-2})$	0.240
Acceptable	1 (Ref.)		1 (Ref.)		1 (Ref.)		1 (Ref.)	
Borderline*	0.94 (0.83–1.07)	0.354	1.07 (0.95–1.20)	0.269	0.98 (0.85–1.11)	0.711	1.00 (0.81–1.24)	0.964
Poor*	1.00 (0.85–1.17)	0.986	1.24 (1.08–1.42)	0.002	0.87 (0.73–1.03)	0.111	0.79 (0.60–1.03)	0.082

Notes: CI, confidence interval; FCS, food consumption score. FCS is continuous data of the food security assessment. Depressive symptoms were defined as CES-D 10 score ≥10. Models are adjusted for age, gender, level of education, marital status, geographical areas of living, smoking habit status, physical activity days, blood pressures, body mass index, diabetes, and cardiovascular diseases. * The exponentiated β-coefficient was used for the logistic models of generalized estimating equation.

4. Discussion

The present study aimed to explore the association between food insecurity and depressive symptoms among adults aged 18–65 years in Indonesia. The borderline and poor food consumption groups represent food insecurity. The present study results suggest that food insecurity was positively significantly associated with depressive symptoms in Indonesian adults. As expected, the secondary findings confirmed that the high prevalence of depressive symptoms occurred among respondents with food insecurity across all ages of adults. Further, the total prevalence rates of food-insecure respondents with depressive symptoms (borderline FCG: 29.3%; poor FCG: 28.1%) was higher than the prevalence rates of food-secure respondents with depressive symptoms (acceptable FCG: 32.1%). The present study's prevalence rates are higher than the national crude prevalence rate of depressive symptoms, which was 3.7% in 2015 [4]. Therefore, the government, health practitioners, and relevant stakeholders need to be more concerned about the issue of food insecurity and depressive symptoms.

One possible action that might help is a food insecurity and depressive symptoms' screening and monitoring process, along with the nutrition health programs for adults. Previous researchers found that the level of education is associated with food insecurity and the increased individual level of stress, which may lead to depressive symptoms [47–49]. Another possible reason is people with less education will more likely experience economic hardship, due to a lower-paid work type or unemployment, which is associated with food insecurity and depressive symptoms [50]. The findings in this study were in line with those of previous research, indicating that the majority of food-insecure respondents had a low level of education and lived in urban areas, with a greater associated risk of economic hardship compared to people with a higher level of education [51].

Moreover, adults who experience a high-burden work type with less income may have depressive symptoms, which can interfere with the ability to manage financial affairs related to food choice and preparation [52,53]. Furthermore, former researchers suggest that unhealthy food choices, for example, Western dietary patterns, which are more likely to contain high calories, high fat, and less diversity, are (partly) associated with depressive symptoms [54,55]. The food consumption score analysis based on the WFP concept is more concerned with the food frequency and quality, and the diversity of diet [25]. One of the explanations is in the food consumption analysis, in which the calculation of food consumption score includes the number of days during which the respondent eats the food type in the FFQ, multiplied by the weight score of each food group type. The highest score refers to all of the food with relatively high energy, good-quality protein, and micronutrients [28]. Therefore, the higher the food consumption score, the better and more diverse the diet and the less food insecurity. However, the present study found that food-insecure respondents had lower food consumption scores than food-secure respondents, indicating that food-insecure respondents possibly consumed lower quality and less diverse food, with high energy and fat density.

Food insecurity is associated with depressive symptoms, overweight and obesity, hypertension, diabetes, and cardiovascular diseases [56–62]. The results of the present study were in line with previous research. The respondents in borderline and poor FCG have lower FCS, and higher body mass index, waist circumference, systolic blood pressure, and CES-D score, than the respondents in the acceptable FCG. One of the reasons to explain the mechanism between food insecurity, overweight, hypertension, and depression is when food-insecure people are unable to choose a properly balanced meal for themselves, and thus eat a low-quality and less diverse diet (high energy, high fat), which eventually leads to being overweight [56]. Food-insecure people are not only at a higher risk of being overweight, but also of increased levels of stress, possibly from a lack of sleep quality due to hunger or worries about providing food the next day [52,63]. On the other hand, continuous food insecurity in a person's life may lead to the onset of depression [11,64]. Pryor and colleagues suggested that food insecurity during young adulthood (18–35 years) co-occurs with three types of mental health problems (i.e., depression, suicidal ideation, and substance use problems in young adulthood) [65].

Furthermore, people with food insecurity are more likely to experience depression and undertake less leisure-time physical activity than those with food security [66–69]. The current study results support the evidence from previous research that the mean of vigorous physical activity (VPA) and moderate physical activity (MPA) days was different between the acceptable FCG (food-secure) and borderline or poor FCG (food-insecure). Moreover, the association between food insecurity and depressive symptoms might be affected by several health factors, which need further exploration using a longitudinal study or more variables. Thus, we further tested the association between food insecurity and depressive symptoms using regression analysis. The results suggested the association was constant even after gradually adjusting for the covariates. The covariates included health and sociodemographic characteristics, such as age, gender, level of education, marital status, geographical area of living, smoking habit status, blood pressure, BMI, incidence of diabetes, and cardiovascular diseases. Taken together, food insecurity was found to have a positive effect on depressive symptoms even after adjustment. The post hoc result showed that respondents aged 40–49 years independently reported levels of poor FCG that were significantly associated with depressive symptoms. The present study results were in line with a previous study that showed that people aged 40–49 are confronted with the most severe problems of food insecurity [18]. The study by Ziliak and Gundersen reported that the "youngest old" suffer from the most severe form of food insecurity compared to those of a younger age or even those over 70 years [70]. The middle-aged food-insecure people might face a recession of income, live in poverty in urban areas, be raising grandchildren, have a limitation on their activities of daily living, or be in a minority [71].

There are several limitations in the present study. First, the dataset that we used was restricted to the selected variables (i.e., the use of the food frequency questionnaire to conduct the food insecurity assessment) for the original study because we used secondary data in this study. However, the FFQ used in this study was widely used from the first wave of the Indonesia Family Life Survey, initiated in 1993, and has also been used in several previous studies [72–74]. Second, the assessment of food insecurity and depressive symptoms was limited to self-reported data. However, the food insecurity measurement from the FFQ was relevant when we defined it from the food frequency and diversity diet [24,25]. Moreover, the use of the CES-D 10 items is widely used to measure the depression or depressive symptoms among adults [30,75]. Third, we could not control for the respondents who received antidepressants or therapy because the IFLS questionnaire did not include a related question. Thus, we suggest future research should further explore the socio-environmental and dietary risk factors of depression and food insecurity. The present study concerns a very important and, at the same time, complex topic of depressive symptoms and lack of food security. These are two public health problems in developing countries that, along with obesity-related non-communicable diseases, significantly affect people's quality of life.

5. Conclusions

To our knowledge, the present study results contribute to the evidence that food insecurity is positively significantly associated with depression symptoms among South-East Asian, particularly Indonesian, adults, as well as for people aged 40–49. Hence, depressive symptoms and food insecurity are public health concerns that need to be improved by health professionals, in conjunction with health and nutrition programs for adults who are at risk of, or currently experiencing, either of these issues. Health professionals must be aware of screening, monitoring, and engaging with food-insecure adults to prevent depression or chronic diseases.

Supplementary Materials: The following are available online at http://www.mdpi.com/2072-6643/11/12/3026/s1, Table S1: One-way ANOVA with Bonferroni Post-Hoc Test Results year 2014, Table S2: One-way ANOVA with Bonferroni Post-Hoc Test Results year 2007.

Author Contributions: E.R.I. and S.-H.Y. conceived and designed the study; E.R.I., H.-Y.F., and Y.-C.C., performed the data analyses; E.R.I., A.C.A., C.-Y.L., Y.-C.C., and S.-H.Y. wrote the paper.

Funding: This research received no external funding.

Acknowledgments: The authors are thankful to the sponsor of this study, Lembaga Pengelola Dana Pendidikan (LPDP), as a part of the author's (Emyr Reisha Isaura) thesis dissertation.

Nutrients **2019**, *11*, 3026

Conflicts of Interest: The authors declare no conflict of interest. The author has presented some part of this study in the Asian Congress of Nutrition 2019, on 4–7 August 2019 at Bali International Convention center, Bali, Indonesia. The funding sponsor had no role in the design of the study; in the collection, analyses, or interpretation of data; in the writing of the manuscript, or in the decision to publish the results.

References

1. Tsai, K.W.; Lin, S.C.; Koo, M. Correlates of depressive symptoms in late middle-aged Taiwanese women: Findings from the 2009 Taiwan National Health Interview Survey. *BMC Womens Health* **2017**, *17*, 103. [CrossRef] [PubMed]

2. National Collaborating Centre for Mental Health. *Depression: The Treatment and Management of Depression in Adults (Updated edition)*; The British Psychological Society and The Royal College of Psychiatrists: Leicester/London, UK, 2010.

3. Marcus, M.; Yasamy, M.T.; van Ommeren, M.V.; Chisholm, D.; Saxena, S. *Depression: A global public health concern*; World Health Organization: Geneva, Switzerland, 2012.

4. World Health Organization. *Depression and Other Common Mental Disorders: Global Health Estimates*; World Health Organization: Geneva, Switzerland, 2017.

5. Brooks, L.K.; Kalyanaraman, N.; Malek, R. Diabetes Care for Patients Experiencing Homelessness: Beyond Metformin and Sulfonylureas. *Am. J. Med.* **2019**, *132*, 408–412. [CrossRef] [PubMed]

6. Ramsey, R.; Giskes, K.; Turrell, G.; Gallegos, D. Food insecurity among adults residing in disadvantaged urban areas: Potential health and dietary consequences. *Public Health Nutr.* **2012**, *15*, 227–237. [CrossRef] [PubMed]

7. Seligman, H.K.; Laraia, B.A.; Kushel, M.B. Food insecurity is associated with chronic disease among low-income NHANES participants. *J. Nutr.* **2010**, *140*, 304–310. [CrossRef] [PubMed]

8. Laraia, B.A. Food insecurity and chronic disease. *Adv. Nutr.* **2013**, *4*, 203–212. [CrossRef] [PubMed]

9. Kim, K.; Frongillo, E.A. Participation in food assistance programs modifies the relation of food insecurity with weight and depression in elders. *J. Nutr.* **2007**, *137*, 1005–1010. [CrossRef]

10. Goldberg, S.L.; Mawn, B.E. Predictors of food insecurity among older adults in the United States. *Public Health Nurs.* **2015**, *32*, 397–407. [CrossRef]

11. Brooks, J.M.; Petersen, C.L.; Titus, A.J.; Umucu, E.; Chiu, C.; Bartels, S.J.; Batsis, J.A. Varying Levels of Food Insecurity Associated with Clinically Relevant Depressive Symptoms in US Adults Aged 60 Years and Over: Results from the 2005–2014 National Health and Nutrition Survey. *J. Nutr. Gerontol. Geriatr.* **2019**, 1–13. [CrossRef]

12. Seligman, H.K.; Schillinger, D. Hunger and socioeconomic disparities in chronic disease. *N. Engl. J. Med.* **2010**, *363*, 6–9. [CrossRef]

13. Seligman, H.K.; Davis, T.C.; Schillinger, D.; Wolf, M.S. Food insecurity is associated with hypoglycemia and poor diabetes self-management in a low-income sample with diabetes. *J. Health Care Poor Underserved* **2010**, *21*, 1227–1233. [CrossRef]

14. Tuthill, E.L.; Sheira, L.A.; Palar, K.; Frongillo, E.A.; Wilson, T.E.; Adedimeji, A.; Merenstein, D.; Cohen, M.H.; Wentz, E.L.; Adimora, A.A.; et al. Persistent Food Insecurity Is Associated with Adverse Mental Health among Women Living with or at Risk of HIV in the United States. *J. Nutr.* **2019**, *149*, 240–248. [CrossRef] [PubMed]

15. Bergmans, R.S.; Zivin, K.; Mezuk, B. Depression, food insecurity and diabetic morbidity: Evidence from the Health and Retirement Study. *J. Psychosom. Res.* **2019**, *117*, 22–29. [CrossRef] [PubMed]

16. Kirkland, J. Food Insecurity and Older Adults. *Res. Public Health* **2019**, *16*, 2294.

17. Burris, M.; Kihlstrom, L.; Arce, K.S.; Prendergast, K.; Dobbins, J.; McGrath, E.; Renda, A.; Shannon, E.; Cordier, T.; Song, Y. Food Insecurity, Loneliness, and Social Support among Older Adults. *J. Hunger Environ. Nutr.* **2019**, 1–16. [CrossRef]

18. Strickhouser, S.; Wright, J.; Donley, A. *Food Insecurity Among Older Adults*; AARP Foundation: Washington DC, USA, 2014.

19. Strauss, J.; Witoelar, F.; Sikoki, B.; Wattie, A.M. *The 4th Wave of the Indonesian Family Life Survey (IFLS4): Overview and Field Report*; WR-675/1-NIA/NICHD; RAND: Santa Monica, CA, USA, 2009.

20. Strauss, J.; Beegel, K.; Sikoki, B.; Dwiyanto, A.; Herawati, Y.; Witoelar, F. *The Third Wave of the Indonesia Family Life Survey: Overview and Field Report*; WR144/1-NIA/NICHD; RAND: Santa Monica, CA, USA, 2004.

21. Strauss, J.; Witoelar, F.; Sikoki, B. *The Fifth Wave of the Indonesia Family Life Survey: Overview and Field Report*; RAND: Santa Monica, CA, USA, 2016.

22. Frankenberg, E.; Karoly, L.A.; Gertler, P.; Achmad, S.; Agung, I.; Hatmadji, S.H.; Sudharto, P. *The 1993 Indonesian Family Life Survey: Overview and Field Report*; RAND: Santa Monica, CA, USA, 1995.

23. Frankenberg, E.; Thomas, D. *The Indonesia Family Life Survey (IFLS): Study Design and Results from Waves 1 and 2*. 2000; DRU2238/1. NIA/NICHD; RAND: Santa Monica, CA, USA, 2000.

24. Hoddinott, J.; Yohannes, Y. Dietary diversity as a food security indicator. *Food Consum. Nutr. Div. Discuss. Pap.* **2002**, *136*, 2002.

25. World Food Programme. *Food Consumption Score Nutritional Quality Analysis Guidelines (FCS-N)*; United Nations World Food Programme, Food Security Analysis (VAM): Rome, Italy, 2015.

26. Wiesmann, D.; Bassett, L.; Benson, T.; Hoddinott, J. *Validation of the World Food Programme s Food Consumption Score and Alternative Indicators of Household Food Security*; IFPRI: Washington, DC, USA, 2009.

27. Isaura, E.R.; Chen, Y.C.; Yang, S.H. Pathways from Food Consumption Score to Cardiovascular Disease: A Seven-Year Follow-Up Study of Indonesian Adults. *Int. J. Environ. Res. Public Health* **2018**, *15*, 1567. [CrossRef]

28. World Food Programme. *Food Consumption Analysis: Calculation and Use of the Food Consumption Score in Food Security Analysis*; World Food Programme: Rome, Italy, 2008.

29. United Nations World Food Programme-Food Security Analysis. *Consolidated Approach to Reporting Indicators of Food Security (CARI) Guidelines*; United Nations World Food Programme, Food security analysis (VAM): Rome, Italy, 2015.

30. Kilburn, K.; Prencipe, L.; Hjelm, L.; Peterman, A.; Handa, S.; Palermo, T. Examination of performance of the Center for Epidemiologic Studies Depression Scale Short Form 10 among African youth in poor, rural households. *BMC Psychiatry* **2018**, *18*, 201. [CrossRef]

31. Andresen, E.M.; Malmgren, J.A.; Carter, W.B.; Patrick, D.L. Screening for depression in well older adults: Evaluation of a short form of the CES-D (Center for Epidemiologic Studies Depression Scale). *Am. J. Prev. Med.* **1994**, *10*, 77–84. [CrossRef]

32. Asante, K.O.; Andoh-Arthur, J. Prevalence and determinants of depressive symptoms among university students in Ghana. *J. Affect. Disord.* **2015**, *171*, 161–166. [CrossRef]

33. Kilburn, K.; Thirumurthy, H.; Halpern, C.T.; Pettifor, A.; Handa, S. Effects of a Large-Scale Unconditional Cash Transfer Program on Mental Health Outcomes of Young People in Kenya. *J. Adolesc. Health* **2016**, *58*, 223–229. [CrossRef]

34. Departemen Kesehatan Republik Indonesia; Direktorat Jenderal Bina Kesehatan Masyarakat; Direktorat Gizi Masyarakat. *Petunjuk Teknis Pemantauan Status Gizi Orang Dewasa Dengan Indeks Massa Tubuh*; Departemen Kesehatan RI: Jakarta, Indonesia, 2003; p. 27.

35. Zeng, Q.; He, Y.; Dong, S.; Zhao, X.; Chen, Z.; Song, Z.; Chang, G.; Yang, F.; Wang, Y. Optimal cut-off values of BMI, waist circumference and waist:height ratio for defining obesity in Chinese adults. *Br. J. Nutr.* **2014**, *112*, 1735–1744. [CrossRef] [PubMed]

36. Bell, K.; Twiggs, J.; Olin, B.R. *Hypertension: The Silent Killer: Updated JNC-8 Guideline Recommendations*; Alabama Pharmacy Association: Montgomery, AL, USA, 2015.

37. Mendis, S.; Puska, P.; Norrving, B. *Global Atlas on Cardiovascular Disease Prevention and Control*; World Health Organization: Geneva, Switzerland, 2011.

38. Liang, K.Y.; Zeger, S.L. Longitudinal data analysis using generalized linear models. *Biometrika* **1986**, *73*, 13–22. [CrossRef]

39. Lipsky, L.M.; Nansel, T.R.; Haynie, D.L.; Liu, D.; Li, K.; Pratt, C.A.; Iannotti, R.J.; Dempster, K.W.; Simons-Morton, B. Diet quality of US adolescents during the transition to adulthood: Changes and predictors. *Am. J. Clin. Nutr.* **2017**, *105*, 1424–1432. [CrossRef] [PubMed]

40. Wang, M. Generalized estimating equations in longitudinal data analysis: A review and recent developments. *Adv. Stat.* **2014**, *2014*, 303728. [CrossRef]

41. Tamers, S.L.; Okechukwu, C.; Bohl, A.A.; Gueguen, A.; Goldberg, M.; Zins, M. The impact of stressful life events on excessive alcohol consumption in the French population: Findings from the GAZEL cohort study. *PLoS ONE* **2014**, *9*, e87653. [CrossRef]

42. Hearst, M.O.; Sirard, J.R.; Lytle, L.; Dengel, D.R.; Berrigan, D. Comparison of 3 measures of physical activity and associations with blood pressure, HDL, and body composition in a sample of adolescents. *J. Phys. Act. Health* **2012**, *9*, 78–85. [CrossRef]

43. Hanley, J.A.; Negassa, A.; Edwardes, M.D.; Forrester, J.E. Statistical analysis of correlated data using generalized estimating equations: An orientation. *Am. J. Epidemiol.* **2003**, *157*, 364–375. [CrossRef]

44. Chen, Y.C.; Tu, Y.K.; Huang, K.C.; Chen, P.C.; Chu, D.C.; Lee, Y.L. Pathway from central obesity to childhood asthma. Physical fitness and sedentary time are leading factors. *Am. J. Respir. Crit. Care Med.* **2014**, *189*, 1194–1203. [CrossRef]

45. Hardin, J.W.; Hilbe, J.M. *Generalized Estimating Equations*, 2nd ed.; CRC Press, Taylor and Francis Group: Boca Raton, FL, USA, 2013.

46. Zeger, S.L.; Liang, K.Y. Longitudinal data analysis for discrete and continuous outcomes. *Biometrics* **1986**, *42*, 121–130. [CrossRef]

47. Laraia, B.A.; Borja, J.B.; Bentley, M.E. Grandmothers, fathers, and depressive symptoms are associated with food insecurity among low-income first-time African-American mothers in North Carolina. *J. Am. Diet Assoc.* **2009**, *109*, 1042–1047. [CrossRef]

48. Laraia, B.A.; Siega-Riz, A.M.; Gundersen, C.; Dole, N. Psychosocial factors and socioeconomic indicators are associated with household food insecurity among pregnant women. *J. Nutr.* **2006**, *136*, 177–182. [CrossRef]

49. Chung, H.K.; Kim, O.Y.; Kwak, S.Y.; Cho, Y.; Lee, K.W.; Shin, M.J. Household Food Insecurity Is Associated with Adverse Mental Health Indicators and Lower Quality of Life among Koreans: Results from the Korea National Health and Nutrition Examination Survey 2012–2013. *Nutrients* **2016**, *8*. [CrossRef] [PubMed]

50. Johnson, C.M.; Sharkey, J.R.; Dean, W.R. Indicators of material hardship and depressive symptoms among homebound older adults living in North Carolina. *J. Nutr. Gerontol. Geriatr.* **2011**, *30*, 154–168. [CrossRef] [PubMed]

51. Sharpe, P.A.; Whitaker, K.; Alia, K.A.; Wilcox, S.; Hutto, B. Dietary Intake, Behaviors and Psychosocial Factors Among Women from Food-Secure and Food-Insecure Households in the United States. *Ethn. Dis.* **2016**, *26*, 139–146. [CrossRef]

52. Leung, C.W.; Epel, E.S.; Willett, W.C.; Rimm, E.B.; Laraia, B.A. Household food insecurity is positively associated with depression among low-income supplemental nutrition assistance program participants and income-eligible nonparticipants. *J. Nutr.* **2015**, *145*, 622–627. [CrossRef] [PubMed]

53. Kuczmarski, M.F.; Cremer Sees, A.; Hotchkiss, L.; Cotugna, N.; Evans, M.K.; Zonderman, A.B. Higher Healthy Eating Index-2005 scores associated with reduced symptoms of depression in an urban population: Findings from the Healthy Aging in Neighborhoods of Diversity Across the Life Span (HANDLS) study. *J. Am. Diet Assoc.* **2010**, *110*, 383–389. [CrossRef] [PubMed]

54. Akbaraly, T.N.; Brunner, E.J.; Ferrie, J.E.; Marmot, M.G.; Kivimaki, M.; Singh-Manoux, A. Dietary pattern and depressive symptoms in middle age. *Br. J. Psychiatry* **2009**, *195*, 408–413. [CrossRef]

55. Le Port, A.; Gueguen, A.; Kesse-Guyot, E.; Melchior, M.; Lemogne, C.; Nabi, H.; Goldberg, M.; Zins, M.; Czernichow, S. Association between dietary patterns and depressive symptoms over time: A 10-year follow-up study of the GAZEL cohort. *PLoS ONE* **2012**, *7*, e51593. [CrossRef]

56. Caamano, M.C.; Garcia, O.P.; Paras, P.; Palacios, J.R.; Rosado, J.L. Overvaluation of Eating and Satiation Explains the Association of Food Insecurity and Food Intake With Obesity and Cardiometabolic Diseases. *Food Nutr. Bull.* **2019**, *1*, 379572119863558. [CrossRef]

57. Weigel, M.M.; Armijos, R.X. Food Insecurity, Cardiometabolic Health, and Health Care in U.S.-Mexico Border Immigrant Adults: An Exploratory Study. *J. Immigr. Minor. Health* **2018**, *21*, 1085–1094. [CrossRef]

58. Morales, M.E.; Berkowitz, S.A. The Relationship between Food Insecurity, Dietary Patterns, and Obesity. *Curr. Nutr. Rep.* **2016**, *5*, 54–60. [CrossRef] [PubMed]

59. Pan, L.; Sherry, B.; Njai, R.; Blanck, H.M. Food insecurity is associated with obesity among US adults in 12 states. *J. Acad. Nutr. Diet* **2012**, *112*, 1403–1409. [CrossRef] [PubMed]

60. Drewnowski, A. Obesity, diets, and social inequalities. *Nutr. Rev.* **2009**, *67*, S36–S39. [CrossRef] [PubMed]

61. Seligman, H.K.; Bindman, A.B.; Vittinghoff, E.; Kanaya, A.M.; Kushel, M.B. Food insecurity is associated with diabetes mellitus: Results from the National Health Examination and Nutrition Examination Survey (NHANES) 1999-2002. *J. Gen. Intern. Med.* **2007**, *22*, 1018–1023. [CrossRef] [PubMed]

62. Drewnowski, A.; Specter, S.E. Poverty and obesity: The role of energy density and energy costs. *Am. J. Clin. Nutr.* **2004**, *79*, 6–16. [CrossRef]

63. Bermudez-Millan, A.; Perez-Escamilla, R.; Segura-Perez, S.; Damio, G.; Chhabra, J.; Osborn, C.Y.; Wagner, J. Psychological Distress Mediates the Association between Food Insecurity and Suboptimal Sleep Quality in Latinos with Type 2 Diabetes Mellitus. *J. Nutr.* **2016**, *146*, 2051–2057. [CrossRef]

64. Polivy, J. Psychological consequences of food restriction. *J. Am. Diet Assoc.* **1996**, *96*, 589–592. [CrossRef]

65. Pryor, L.; Lioret, S.; van der Waerden, J.; Fombonne, E.; Falissard, B.; Melchior, M. Food insecurity and mental health problems among a community sample of young adults. *Soc. Psychiatry Psychiatr. Epidemiol.* **2016**, *51*, 1073–1081. [CrossRef]

66. Holtermann, A.; Krause, N.; Van der Beek, A.J.; Straker, L. The physical activity paradox: Six reasons why occupational physical activity (OPA) does not confer the cardiovascular health benefits that leisure time physical activity does. *Br. J. Sports Med.* **2018**, *52*, 149–150. [CrossRef]

67. Liu, Y.; Shu, X.O.; Wen, W.; Saito, E.; Rahman, M.S.; Tsugane, S.; Tamakoshi, A.; Xiang, Y.B.; Yuan, J.M.; Gao, Y.T.; et al. Association of leisure-time physical activity with total and cause-specific mortality: A pooled analysis of nearly a half million adults in the Asia Cohort Consortium. *Int. J. Epidemiol.* **2018**, *47*, 771–779. [CrossRef]

68. Liu, X.; Zhang, D.; Liu, Y.; Sun, X.; Han, C.; Wang, B.; Ren, Y.; Zhou, J.; Zhao, Y.; Shi, Y.; et al. Dose-Response Association Between Physical Activity and Incident Hypertension: A Systematic Review and Meta-Analysis of Cohort Studies. *Hypertension* **2017**, *69*, 813–820. [CrossRef]

69. Hamer, M.; Molloy, G.J.; de Oliveira, C.; Demakakos, P. Leisure time physical activity, risk of depressive symptoms, and inflammatory mediators: The English Longitudinal Study of Ageing. *Psychoneuroendocrinology* **2009**, *34*, 1050–1055. [CrossRef]

70. Ziliak, J.P.; Gundersen, C. *The State of Senior Hunger in America 2014: An Annual Report*; National Foundation to End Senior Hunger: Alexandria, VA, USA, 2013.

71. Ziliak, J.P.; Gundersen, C. *Food Insecurity Among Older Adults*; AARP: Washington, DC, USA, 2011.

72. Isaura, E.R.; Chen, Y.C.; Yang, S.H. The Association of Food Consumption Scores, Body Shape Index, and Hypertension in a Seven-Year Follow-Up among Indonesian Adults: A Longitudinal Study. *Int. J. Environ. Res. Public Health* **2018**, *15*, 175. [CrossRef] [PubMed]

73. Hussain, M.A.; Mamun, A.A.; Reid, C.; Huxley, R.R. Prevalence, Awareness, Treatment and Control of Hypertension in Indonesian Adults Aged >/=40 Years: Findings from the Indonesia Family Life Survey (IFLS). *PLoS ONE* **2016**, *11*, e0160922. [CrossRef]

74. Vaezghasemi, M.; Razak, F.; Ng, N.; Subramanian, S.V. Inter-individual inequality in BMI: An analysis of Indonesian Family Life Surveys (1993-2007). *SSM Popul. Health* **2016**, *2*, 876–888. [CrossRef]

75. James, C.; Powell, M.; Seixas, A.; Bateman, A.; Pengpid, S.; Peltzer, K. Exploring the psychometric properties of the CES-D-10 and its practicality in detecting depressive symptomatology in 27 low- and middle-income countries. *Int. J. Psychol.* **2019**. [CrossRef]

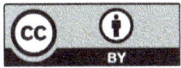

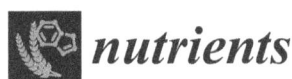 *nutrients*

Review

Microbiota-Orientated Treatments for Major Depression and Schizophrenia

Guillaume B. Fond [1,*], Jean-Christophe Lagier [2], Stéphane Honore [1], Christophe Lancon [1], Théo Korchia [1], Pierre-Louis Sunhary De Verville [1], Pierre-Michel Llorca [3], Pascal Auquier [1], Eric Guedj [4] and Laurent Boyer [1]

[1] Hôpitaux Universitaires de Marseille, Department de Psychiatrie Universitaire, EA 3279: Aix-Marseille Université, CEReSS—Health Service Research and Quality of Life Center, 27 Boulevard Jean Moulin, 13005 Marseille, France; stephane.honore@ap-hm.fr (S.H.); christophe.lancon@ap-hm.fr (C.L.); theo.korchia@ap-hm.fr (T.K.); deverville.pierrelouis@gmail.com (P.-L.S.D.V.); pascal.auquier@univ-amu.fr (P.A.); laurent.boyer@ap-hm.fr (L.B)
[2] Aix Marseille University, Institut de Recherche pour le Développement, Microbes Evolution Phylogeny and Infection, Assistance Publique Hôpitaux de Marseille, Institut Hospitalo Universitaire Méditerranée Infection, 13005 Marseille, France; JeanChristophe.LAGIER@ap-hm.fr
[3] CHU de Clermont-Ferrand, F-63000 Cllermont-Ferrand, France; pmllorca@chu-clermontferrand.fr
[4] Aix-Marseille Université, CNRS, Ecole Centrale de Marseille, UMR 7249, Institut Fresnel, Département de médecine nucléaire, CERIMED, Aix-Marseille Université, F-13005 Marseille, France; eric.guedj@ap-hm.fr
*   Correspondence: guillaume.fond@gmail.com

Received: 7 February 2020; Accepted: 2 April 2020; Published: 8 April 2020

Abstract: Background and significance. There is a need to develop new hypothesis-driven treatment for both both major depression (MD) and schizophrenia in which the risk of depression is 5 times higher than the general population. Major depression has been also associated with poor illness outcomes including pain, metabolic disturbances, and less adherence. Conventional antidepressants are partly effective, and 44% of the subjects remain unremitted under treatment. Improving MD treatment efficacy is thus needed to improve the SZ prognosis. Microbiota-orientated treatments are currently one of the most promising tracks. Method. This work is a systematic review synthetizing data of arguments to develop microbiota-orientated treatments (including fecal microbiota transplantation (FMT)) in major depression and schizophrenia. Results. The effectiveness of probiotic administration in MD constitutes a strong evidence for developing microbiota-orientated treatments. Probiotics have yielded medium-to-large significant effects on depressive symptoms, but it is still unclear if the effect is maintained following probiotic discontinuation. Several factors may limit MD improvement when using probiotics, including the small number of bacterial strains administered in probiotic complementary agents, as well as the presence of a disturbed gut microbiota that probably limits the probiotics' impact. FMT is a safe technique enabling to improve microbiota in several gut disorders. The benefit/risk ratio of FMT has been discussed and has been recently improved by capsule administration. Conclusion. Cleaning up the gut microbiota by transplanting a totally new human gut microbiota in one shot, which is referred to as FMT, is likely to strongly improve the efficacy of microbiota-orientated treatments in MD and schizophrenia and maintain the effect over time. This hypothesis should be tested in future clinical trials.

Keywords: psychiatry; schizophrenia; depression; microbiota; transplantation

1. Introduction

Major depression (MD) is described as "a global crisis" by the World Health Organization (WHO) [1]. Major depression can affect anyone from young people to seniors, and it is one of the most widespread illnesses, often co-existing with other serious illnesses [2]. According to the WHO, MD was ranked as the third leading cause of the global burden of disease in 2004 and will likely have moved to the first place by 2030 [3]. It is now estimated that 350 million people are affected by MD worldwide, which poses a significant health and economic burden to society [4–6]. In 2016, MD was the first source of disability, accounting for 1059 worldwide disability-adjusted life years (DALYs)/100,000 habitants, thereby noticeably preceding ischemic and hemorrhagic stroke (787 and 923 respectively), hypertensive heart disease (242), Alzheimer disease (470), cancers (liver (295), colon (249), breast (208), and HIV (169)) [7]. Major depression was responsible for 48.7% of all worldwide DALYs related to mental and substance use disorders [7]. This alarming figure is a wakeup call for researchers and should encourage them to address this global non-communicable disease.

Major depression is heterogeneous and improving its treatment may require isolating more specific subgroups in the so-called precision medicine approach. Major depressionv has been identified as a frequent comorbidity of other major psychiatric disorders including schizophrenia (SZ). A half of SZ patients have been identified with MD that has been associated with impaired quality of life which suggests a 5 times higher risk of MD in this population compared to non-SZ individuals. Yet MD remains poorly diagnosed and poorly treated in this population [8–10]. Some studies suggest that MD-SZ may be different from non-SZ MD with lower placebo response and higher impact on functioning [9,11–13]. Major depression in schizophrenia (MD-SZ) has been also associated with other poor illness outcomes including pain, metabolic disturbances, less adherence and lower quality of life [8,14,15]. Treating depression is thus needed to improve the SZ prognosis [16]. Conventional antidepressants are partly effective, but 44% of the subjects remain unremitted under treatment [9]. Yet, funding for research directed to improving diagnosis and treatment of MD-SZ is sadly lacking [17].

Though conventional treatments have improved MD prognosis, they still remain unsatisfactory. The response rate of antidepressants amounts to only 17.7% in the general population [18]. An explanation for this high rate of non-response and relapses relies on the observation that current pharmacological treatments are primarily based on the monoaminergic hypothesis, without involving the personalized medicine approach. According to this hypothesis, MD is principally due to the fact of a deficit of three neurotransmitters in the brain (i.e., serotonin, norepinephrine, and dopamine). All current antidepressants target serotonin, norepinephrine, or dopamine deficits. The high rate of therapeutic failure in psychiatry can most likely be accounted for by the limitations pertaining to brain-orientated treatments. Current treatments do improve neurotransmitters deficits, yet without addressing the source of these deficits. This may explain the high relapsing rates and chronic illness course.

The key to breaking the deadlock of SZ-MD treatment may be found in the intestinal microbiota [19]. The links between gut microbiota disturbances and brain dysfunction have clearly been demonstrated in rodents. The so-called "gut-brain axis" has already been extensively described in humans with six pathways [19,20]: vagal nerve stimulation; inflammation and cytokine modulation; decreased gut permeability; short-chain fatty acid and neurotransmitter synthesis; nutrient absorption; Hypothalamic–pituitary–adrenal (HPA) stress axis (cortisol) modulation (Figure 1). Moreover, microbiota dysfunctions have been associated with peripheral immune inflammation as well as neuro-inflammation (also called microglia activation) [21].

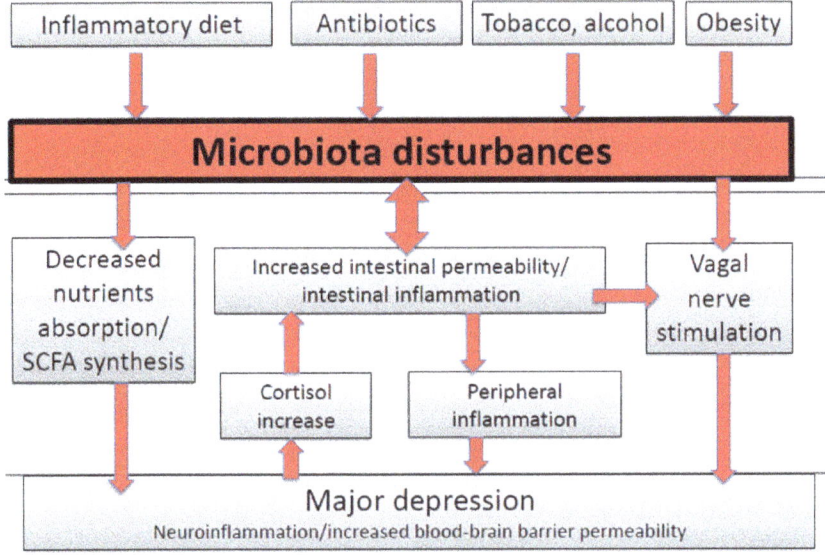

Figure 1. The gut–brain axis in major depression.

Several clues indicate that targeting microbiota may be particularly relevant in schizophrenia (SZ). Schizophrenia patients are treated by antipsychotics that induce gastrointestinal disorders (including constipation) that may impact their gut microbiota. More than one quarter of SZ stabilized outpatients have abdominal obesity, which is a clinical marker of disturbed microbiota, and MD has been found to be the best predictor of rapid high weight gain in SZ [14]. Abnormal bacterial markers have been identified in the blood of SZ patients [22,23]. Emerging data show that about 30% of SZ people have elevated antigliadin antibodies (AGA) of the IgG type, representing a possible subgroup of schizophrenia patients with increased gut permeability [24]. Also, recent data have shown a high correlation of IgG-mediated antibodies between the periphery and cerebral spinal fluid in schizophrenia but not healthy controls, particularly AGA IgG suggesting that these antibodies may be crossing the blood-brain barrier with resulting neuroinflammation [25]. Schizophrenia has been extensively associated with other abnormal translational markers, suggesting an increased gut permeability in this illness [23,25–29]. More than one in five SZ patients are identified with metabolic syndrome [30], and one-third with chronic low-grade peripheral inflammation [31–34]. This inflammation is a good marker of central inflammation and has also been associated with SZ-MD [35].

Our hypothesis is that replacing the whole microbiota of SZ-MD patients (the so-called fecal microbiota transplantation (FMT)) may improve their mental and physical health, and more specifically their depressive symptoms and quality of life. Schizophrenia combined with MD and/or inflammation may be a target of choice for microbiota-orientated therapies.

The objective was to synthetize current data for testing microbiota-orientated treatments and to explore the benefit/risk ratio of FMT in major depression and schizophrenia.

2. Methods

This meta-analysis was based on the Preferred Reporting Items for Systematic reviews and Meta-Analysis (PRISMA) criteria [36] (Figure 1). Medline®database was explored from its inception to March, 22th 2020 without language restriction. The research paradigm was: (depression OR schizophrenia) AND (gut microbiota). The references of each article were also checked. Medline is considered as the database of highest quality level. The associated articles were also explored.

Scopus®and ScienceDirect®databases were explored with the same strategy (limited to research articles and research reviews and human studies). Two reviewers (GF and LB) decided on eligibility and extracted data from included studies. As this review involved data from published studies, an institutional review board approval was not required.

2.1. Criteria for Included Studies:

- Design: Human observational and interventional studies and meta-analyses including human data;
- Exploring the association between microbiota disturbances (or irritable bowel syndrome) and major depression or schizophrenia defined by a DSM or ICD-based diagnostic tool (structured clinical interview) OR assessing the efficacy of a microbiota-orientated therapy (probiotics or fecal microbiota transplantation).

2.2. Exclusion Criteria:

- animal studies;
- studies including no individuals with major depression or schizophrenia;
- case reports;
- reviews.

3. Results

Fourteen studies were included in the present review.

3.1. Microbiota-Orientated Therapies and Their Interest for Major Depression

Irritable bowel syndrome is considered as a paradigmatic microbiota-induced illness. We have published a meta-analysis suggesting that patients with irritable bowel syndrome were at higher risk of major depression [37], confirming the potential causal or bilateral relationship between microbiota disturbances and major depression. Several studies have shown microbiota disturbances in patients with major depression; these disturbances are summarized in Table 1 [38–50].

Table 1. Human studies exploring microbiota disturbances in major depression and the interest of microbiota-orientated therapies.

Author/Date	Sample Size and Study Population (N)	Techniques	Major Findings	Interpretation
Fond et al. 2014 [37]	10 studies (885 patients and 1384 HCs)	Meta-analysis	Patients with IBS had significant higher anxiety and depression levels than controls (respectively, SMD = 0.76, 95% CI 0.47; 0.69, $p < 0.01$, I2 = 81.7% and SMD = 0.80, 95% CI 0.42; 1.19, $p < 0.01$, I2 = 90.7%). This significant difference was confirmed for patients with IBS-C and -D subtypes for anxiety, and only in IBS-D patients for depression.	Patients with IBS had significantly higher levels of anxiety and depression than HCs.
Liu et al. 2019 [51]	29 studies involving 3088 participants	Meta-analysis	Prebiotics did not differ from placebo for depression (d = −0.08, $p = 0.51$) or anxiety (d = 0.12, $p = 0.11$). Probiotics yielded small but significant effects for depression (d = −0.24, $p < 0.01$) and anxiety (d = −0.10, $p = 0.03$). Sample type was a moderator for probiotics and depression, with a larger effect observed for clinical/medical samples (d = −0.45, $p < 0.001$) than community ones. This effect increased to medium-to-large in a preliminary analysis restricted to psychiatric samples (d = −0.73, $p < 0.001$).	There is general support for antidepressant and anxiolytic effects of probiotics, but the pooled effects were reduced by the paucity of trials with clinical samples.
Ng et al. 2019 [49]	3 studies	Meta-analysis	No significant difference in schizophrenia symptoms between the group that received probiotic supplementation and the placebo group post-intervention as the standardized mean difference was -0.0884 (95% CI -0.380 to 0.204, $p = 0.551$). Separate analyses were performed to investigate the effect of probiotic supplementation on positive or negative symptoms of schizophrenia alone. In both instances, no significant difference was observed as well.	Based on current evidence, limited inferences can be made regarding the efficacy of probiotics in schizophrenia
Kiecolt-Glaser et al. 2018 [50]	43 (N = 86) healthy married couples, ages 24–61 (mean = 38.22)	Translocation of bacterial endotoxin (lipopolysaccharide, LPS) from the gut microbiota	Participants with more hostile marital interactions had higher LPS-binding protein (LBP) than those who were less hostile. Additionally, the combination of more hostile marital interactions with a mood disorder history was associated with higher LBP/sCD14 ratios.	The combination of more hostile marital interactions with a mood disorder history was associated with higher LBP/sCD14 ratios.

Table 1. *Cont.*

Author/Date	Sample Size and Study Population (N)	Techniques	Major Findings	Interpretation
Chen et al. 2018 [44,45]	10 patients (age: 18–56 years, five women) who had MDD and 10 HCs (age: 24–65 years, five women) matched for sex, age, and BMI	Comparative metaproteomics analysis on the basis of an isobaric tag for relative and absolute quantification coupled with tandem mass spectrometry	279 significantly differentiated bacterial proteins ($p <$ 0.05) were detected and used for further bioinformatic analysis. According to phylogenetic analysis, statistically significant differences were observed for four phyla: *Bacteroidetes*, *Proteobacteria*, *Firmicutes*, *Actinobacteria* ($p <$ 0.05, for each). Abundances of 16 bacterial families were significantly different between the MDD and healthy controls ($p < 0.05$). Cluster of Orthologous Groups analysis and Kyoto Encyclopedia of Genes and Genomes pathway analysis showed that disordered metabolic pathways of bacterial proteins were mainly involved in glucose metabolism and amino acid metabolism.	Fecal microbiota signatures were altered significantly in MDD patients.
Peter et al. 2018 [38]	48 patients with IBS (Rome III criteria, M (SD) age = 42 (15) years, 35 female, 25 diarrhea-dominant, 5 constipation-dominant, and 18 alternating-type IBS)	alpha and beta diversity, correlational analyses of bacterial abundance and comparisons among subgroups defined by thresholds of psychological and IBS symptom variables, and machine learning to identify bacterial patterns corresponding with psychological distress.	Thirty-one patients (65%) showed elevated psychological distress, 22 (31%) anxiety, and 10 depression (21%). Microbial beta diversity was significantly associated with distress and depression (q = 0.036 each, q values are p values false discovery rate-corrected for multiple testing). Depression was negatively associated with *Lachnospiraceae* abundance (Spearman's $\varrho = -0.58$, q = 0.018). Patients exceeding thresholds of distress, anxiety, depression, and stress perception showed significantly higher abundances of *Proteobacteria* (q = 0.020–0.036). Patients with anxiety were characterized by elevated *Bacteroidaceae* (q = 0.036). A signature of 148 unclassified species accounting for 3.9% of total bacterial abundance co-varied systematically with the presence of psychological distress.	Psychological variables significantly segregated gut microbial features, underscoring the role of brain-gut-microbiota interaction in IBS. A microbial signature corresponding with psychological distress was identified.

Table 1. *Cont.*

Author/Date	Sample Size and Study Population (N)	Techniques	Major Findings	Interpretation
Kelly et al. 2016 [39]	34 MDD patients and 33 matched HCs	16s rRNA sequencing	Chao1 richness (U = 424, p = 0.005), total observed species (U = 441, p = 0.002) and phylogenetic diversity (U = 447.5, p = 0.001) were decreased in the depressed group. was no difference in Shannon diversity (U = 350, p = 0.197). Significant differences in beta diversity between the healthy and depressed groups (Bray-Curtis (p = 0.014), unweighted unifrac (p = 0.002) and weighted unifrac (p = 0.018) were unable to separate groups according to PCoA analysis). The difference of the global microbiota composition from the 16S rRNA data of the depressed and control groups was assessed by ordination. Statistics based on random permutations of the redundancy analysis (RDA) showed that the depressed group is significantly separated at genus level (p = 0.03) from the control group. No difference on intestinal permeability, short chain fatty acids, fecal metabolites has been reported.	Depression is associated with decreased gut microbiota richness and diversity
Lin et al. 2017 [48]	N = 10 MDD	V3–V4 region of the 16S rRNA gene was extracted from the fecal microbial communities in MDD patients, PCR amplified and sequenced on the Illumina Miseq platform	More phylum Firmicutes, less Bacteroidetes, and more genus Prevotella, Klebsiella, Streptococcus and Clostridium XI were found in MDD patients. The changes of the proportion of Prevotella and Klebsiella were consistent with Hamilton depression rating scale.	Prevotella and Klebsiella proportion in fecal microbial communities should be concerned in the diagnosis and therapeutic monitoring of MDD in future.
Liu et al. 2016 [42]	N = 100 40 with diarrhea-predominant IBS (IBS-D), 15 with depression, 25 with comorbidities of depression and IBS patients, and 20 healthy individuals (controls)	Colonic mucosal inflammation was assayed by immunohistochemical analyses of sigmoid biopsied tissues	Fecal microbiota signatures were similar between patients with IBS-D and depression presented, in that they were less diverse than samples from controls and had similar abundances of alterations. were characterized by high proportions of *Bacteroides* (Type I), *Prevotella* (Type II), or non-dominant microbiota (Type III). Most patients with IBS-D or depression had Type I or Type II profiles (IBS-D had 85% Type I and Type II, depression had 80% Type I and Type II profiles).	Patients with IBS-D and depression have similar alterations in fecal microbiota; these might be related to the pathogenesis of these disorders. 3 microbial profiles in patients could indicate different subtypes of IBS and depression or be used as diagnostic biomarkers

Table 1. *Cont.*

Author/Date	Sample Size and Study Population (N)	Techniques	Major Findings	Interpretation
Jiang et al. 2015 [43]	46 patients with depression (29 active-MDD and 17 responded-MDD) and 30 healthy controls (HCs).	high-throughput pyrosequencing	Increased fecal bacterial α-diversity was found in the active-MDD (a-MDD) vs. the HC group but not in the responded-MDD (R-MDD) vs. the HC group. *Bacteroidetes*, *Proteobacteria*, and *Actinobacteria* strongly increased in level, whereas that of *Firmicutes* was significantly reduced in the A-MDD and R-MDD groups compared with the HC group. Despite profound interindividual variability, levels of several predominant genera were significantly different between the MDD and HC groups. Most notably, the MDD groups had increased levels of *Enterobacteriaceae* and *Alistipes* but reduced levels of *Faecalibacterium*. A negative correlation was observed between *Faecalibacterium* and the severity of depressive symptoms.	These findings enable a better understanding of changes in the fecal microbiota composition in such patients, showing either a predominance of some potentially harmful bacterial groups or a reduction in beneficial bacterial genera.
Kleiman et al. 2015 [41]	Inpatients with anorexia nervosa at admission (T1; $n = 16$) and discharge (T2; $n = 10$). Patients with anorexia nervosa were compared with healthy individuals who participated in a previous study (HCs).	Genomic DNA was isolated from stool samples, and bacterial composition was characterized by 454 pyrosequencing of the 16S rRNA gene.	Significant changes emerged between T1 and T2 in taxa abundance and beta (between-sample) diversity of patients with anorexia nervosa. Patients with anorexia nervosa had significantly lower alpha (within-sample) diversity than did HCs at both T1 ($p = 0.0001$) and T2 ($p = 0.016$), and differences in taxa abundance were found between anorexia nervosa patients and HCs.	There was evidence of an intestinal dysbiosis in anorexia nervosa and an association between mood and the enteric microbiota in this patient population
Madan et al. 2020 [47]	Adult MDD inpatients (N = 111)	16S rRNA gene sequencing and whole genome shotgun sequencing	Depression and anxiety severity shortly after admission were negatively associated with bacterial richness and alpha diversity. Additional analyses revealed a number of bacterial taxa associated with depression and anxiety severity. Gut microbiota richness and alpha diversity early in the course of hospitalization was a significant predictor of depression remission at discharge.	There is a gut microbiota relationship with symptom severity among MDD inpatients as well as a relationship to remission of depression post-treatment.

Table 1. *Cont.*

Author/Date	Sample Size and Study Population (N)	Techniques	Major Findings	Interpretation
Mason et al. 2020 [46]	N = 70 (60 psychiatric subjects; MDD (comorbid with anxiety), n = 38, anxiety only, n = 8, MDD only without anxiety, n = 14, HCs n = 10	Quantitative PCR and 16S rRNA sequencing	Altered microbiota correlated with pre-defined clinical presentation, with *Bacteroides* (p = 0.011) and the *Clostridium leptum* subgroup (p = 0.023) significantly different between clinical categories. Cluster analysis of the total sample using weighted UniFrac β-diversity of the gut microbiota identified two different clusters defined by differences in bacterial distribution. Cluster 2 had higher *Bacteroides* (p = 0.006), and much reduced presence of *Clostridiales* (p < 0.001) compared to Cluster 1. *Bifidobacterium* (p = 0.0173) was also reduced in Cluster 2 compared to Cluster 1. When evaluated for clinical charateristics, anhedonia scores in Cluster 2 were higher than in Cluster 1.	Reduced or absent *Clostridia* was consistently seen in those with depression, independent of the presence of anxiety. Conversely, reduced *Bacteroides* may be more associated with the presence of anxiety, independent of the presence of depression.
Naseribafrouei et al., 2014 [40]	N = 55 (37 MDD, and 18 HCs)	Illumina deep sequencing of 16S rRNA gene amplicons	The order *Bacteroidales* showed an overrepresentation (p = 0.05), while the family *Lachnospiracae* showed an underrepresentation (p = 0.02) of Operational Taxonomic Units associated with depression.	Several correlations were found between depression and fecal microbiota.

MDD: Major depressive disorder. IBS: irritable bowel syndrome. HCs: Healthy controls. BMI: body mass index.

The effectiveness of probiotic administration in MD constitutes a strong evidence for developing microbiota-orientated treatments in this indication. Probiotics have yielded medium-to-large significant effects in the setting of depression (d = −0.73 (95% CI = −1.02−−0.44)) in a recent meta-analysis [51]. Approximately half of all existing studies were published over the past two years, reflecting the rapidly growing interest in this area. At the time of this submission, 29 studies involving 3088 participants were published so far. Duration of probiotic administration across trials ranged from 8 days to 45 weeks, whereas it is still unclear if the effect is maintained following probiotic discontinuation.

Two factors may limit MD improvement when probiotics are administered: (1) the small number of bacterial strains administered in probiotic complementary agents (often only one to five bacterial strains including *Lactobacilli*, either alone or in combination with *Bifidobacterium*), and (2) the presence of a disturbed gut microbiota that limits probiotics' efficacy (the so-called gut microbiota "resilience"). Cleaning up the gut microbiota and transplanting a totally new human gut microbiota in one shot (the so-called fecal microbiota transplantation) would thus strongly improve the effect size.

3.2. Fecal Microbiota Transplantation's Effectiveness in Non-Psychiatric Diseases

If MD is actually associated with microbiota dysfunctions, replacing disturbed microbiota by a healthy one appears to be one of the most promising approach to improve MD [52]. FMT has been described as "the ultimate probiotic" as it provides an entire microbiome to the recipient. This therapy delivers a much greater number and diversity of bacteria than any current commercially available preparation. In the past decade, there has been a heightened interest in the use of this therapy [53], predominantly driven by increasing rates of recurrent *Clostridium difficile* infection [54–56].

This procedure was proven associated with 87%–100% clinical resolution of recurrent or refractory *C. difficile* infections [56–60]. This impressive success rate is presumably due to the ability of the transplanted bacteria to recolonize/occupy the missing components/niches of the normal intestinal microbiota thus removing the microbial niche that *C. difficile* would otherwise exploit.

In addition to this main application, FMT has demonstrated promising results in other diseases as well such as ulcerative colitis [61,62] or inflammatory bowel diseases [63].

3.3. Fecal Microbiota Transplantation's Safety in Non-Psychiatric Diseases

No serious adverse event related to FMT has been reported in the literature. In a recent review, the commonest FMT-attributable adverse event was abdominal discomfort, which was reported in 19 publications [64].

There is a potential to transmit infection via contaminated donor stool. The donor stool must therefore undergo microscopy and culture for potential bacterial pathogens, microscopy for ova, cysts and parasites as well as viral studies and C. *difficile* toxin analysis. Blood testing to exclude HIV, Hepatitis B and C and syphilis must be undertaken.

Changes in fecal microbiota have been found in patients with a number gastrointestinal and extra-intestinal diseases. Changes in the microbiome of patients with inflammatory bowel diseases and irritable bowel syndrome are well documented in the literature [65].

There have also been associations between various bowel flora, obesity, and the metabolic syndrome. The association has not been documented as causal, and it appears probably related to the diet consumed by these subjects. It would, however, be prudent to exclude donors with the metabolic syndrome.

SZ patients are already treated with antipsychotics, antidepressants, and other psychotropic drugs that have many side-effects (including sedation, weight gain, neurological disorders, diarrhea, and constipation), the FMT appears as a safe treatment in comparison of the standard treatment for SZ and MD. The risk–benefit balance seems favorable.

3.4. Oral Capsules Administration: An Improvement for Fecal Microbiota Transplantation Safety

The oral capsule administration form has proven an equal effectiveness [66] and will prevent the adverse event due to the conventional colonoscopy-delivered upper and lower gastrointestinal routes of FMT, especially bowel perforation over-sedation, aspiration, bleeding, and splenic laceration [67,68]. Some studies reported patient deaths due to the underlying disease, where the patient has not responded to the FMT. Our clinical experience and our 5 years collaboration with patients' associations has also shown to us that an important rate of the patients and their relatives are waiting for innovating treatments targeting new pathways, with a better tolerance than antipsychotics. In France, the microbiota hypothesis is very popular and highly broadcasted in the media.

4. Conclusions

Cleaning up the gut microbiota by transplanting a totally new human gut microbiota in one shot, which is referred to as FMT, is likely to strongly improve the efficacy and maintains the effect over time. The safety and acceptability have been recently improved with capsule administration that should be evaluated in future clinical trials for the treatment of major depression and schizophrenia. Future trials should confirm the effectiveness and identify responder profiles in the context of personalized medicine.

Author Contributions: Conceptualization, G.B.F., J.-C.L. and L.B.; methodology, G.B.F.; resources, G.B.F.; data curation, G.B.F.; writing—original draft preparation, G.B.F., J.-C.L. and L.B.; writing—review and editing, G.B.F., J.-C.L., L.B., S.H., C.L., T.K., P.-L.S.D.V., P.-M.L., P.A., E.G.; supervision L.B.; funding acquisition, G.B.F. and L.B. All authors have read and agreed to the published version of the manuscript.

Funding: This work was funded by Hôpitaux Universitaires de Marseille (HUM), grant number AORC-2018.

Conflicts of Interest: The authors declare no conflict of interest.

References

1. WHO. *Depression: A Global Crisis. World Mental Health Day, October 10 2012*; World Federation for Mental Health: Occoquan, VA, USA, 2012.
2. Fond, G.; Lancon, C.; Auquier, P.; Boyer, L. Prevalence of major depression in France in the general population and in specific populations from 2000 to 2018: A systematic review of the literature. *Presse Med. Paris Fr. 1983* **2019**, *48*, 365–375.
3. Fond, G.; Masson, M.; Auquier, P.; Da Fonseca, D.; Lançon, C.; Llorca, P.-M.; Boyer, L. The key role of psychiatry in the development of French health-related sustainable development goals. *L'Encephale* **2019**, *45*, 99–100. [CrossRef] [PubMed]
4. Sobocki, P.; Jönsson, B.; Angst, J.; Rehnberg, C. Cost of depression in Europe. *J. Ment. Health Policy Econ.* **2006**, *9*, 87–98. [PubMed]
5. Greenberg, P.E.; Fournier, A.-A.; Sisitsky, T.; Pike, C.T.; Kessler, R.C. The economic burden of adults with major depressive disorder in the United States (2005 and 2010). *J. Clin. Psychiatry* **2015**, *76*, 155–162. [CrossRef] [PubMed]
6. Fond, G.; Masson, M.; Lançon, C.; Auquier, P.; Boyer, L. Updating of the French recommendations for the first-line treatment of major depression. *L'Encephale* **2019**, *45*, 457–458. [CrossRef]
7. Hay, S.I.; Abajobir, A.A.; Abate, K.H.; Abbafati, C.; Abbas, K.M.; Abd-Allah, F.; Abdulkader, R.S.; Abdulle, A.M.; Abebo, T.A.; Abera, S.F.; et al. GBD 2016 DALYs and HALE Collaborators Global, regional, and national disability-adjusted life-years (DALYs) for 333 diseases and injuries and healthy life expectancy (HALE) for 195 countries and territories, 1990–2016: A systematic analysis for the global burden of disease study 2016. *Lancet Lond. Engl.* **2017**, *390*, 1260–1344.
8. Andrianarisoa, M.; Boyer, L.; Godin, O.; Brunel, L.; Bulzacka, E.; Aouizerate, B.; Berna, F.; Capdevielle, D.; Dorey, J.M.; Dubertret, C.; et al. Childhood trauma, depression and negative symptoms are independently associated with impaired quality of life in schizophrenia. Results from the national FACE-SZ cohort. *Schizophr. Res.* **2017**, *185*, 173–181. [CrossRef]

9. Fond, G.; Boyer, L.; Berna, F.; Godin, O.; Bulzacka, E.; Andrianarisoa, M.; Brunel, L.; Aouizerate, B.; Capdevielle, D.; Chereau, I.; et al. Remission of depression in patients with schizophrenia and comorbid major depressive disorder: Results from the FACE-SZ cohort. *Br. J. Psychiatry* **2018**, *213*, 464–470. [CrossRef]

10. Alessandrini, M.; Lançon, C.; Fond, G.; Faget-Agius, C.; Richieri, R.; Faugere, M.; Metairie, E.; Boucekine, M.; Llorca, P.-M.; Auquier, P.; et al. A structural equation modelling approach to explore the determinants of quality of life in schizophrenia. *Schizophr. Res.* **2016**, *171*, 27–34. [CrossRef]

11. Fond, G.; Godin, O.; Dumontaud, M.; Faget, C.; Schürhoff, F.; Berna, F.; Aouizerate, B.; Capdevielle, D.; Chereau, I.; D'Amato, T.; et al. Sexual dysfunctions are associated with major depression, chronic inflammation and anticholinergic consumption in the real-world schizophrenia FACE-SZ national cohort. *Prog. Neuropsychopharmacol. Biol. Psychiatry* **2019**, *94*, 109654. [CrossRef]

12. Kucerova, J.; Babinska, Z.; Horska, K.; Kotolova, H. The common pathophysiology underlying the metabolic syndrome, schizophrenia and depression. A review. *Biomed. Pap. Med. Fac. Univ. Palacký Olomouc Czechoslov.* **2015**, *159*, 208–214. [CrossRef] [PubMed]

13. Gregory, A.; Mallikarjun, P.; Upthegrove, R. Treatment of depression in schizophrenia: Systematic review and meta-analysis. *Br. J. Psychiatry J. Ment. Sci.* **2017**, *211*, 198–204. [CrossRef] [PubMed]

14. Godin, O.; Leboyer, M.; Schürhoff, F.; Boyer, L.; Andrianarisoa, M.; Brunel, L.; Bulzacka, E.; Aouizerate, B.; Berna, F.; Capdevielle, D.; et al. Predictors of rapid high weight gain in schizophrenia: Longitudinal analysis of the French FACE-SZ cohort. *J. Psychiatr. Res.* **2017**, *94*, 62–69. [CrossRef] [PubMed]

15. Fond, G.; Boyer, L.; Andrianarisoa, M.; Godin, O.; Bulzacka, E.; Berna, F.; Brunel, L.; Coulon, N.; Aouizerate, B.; Capdevielle, D.; et al. Self-reported pain in patients with schizophrenia. Results from the national first-step FACE-SZ cohort. *Prog. Neuropsychopharmacol. Biol. Psychiatry* **2018**, *85*, 62–68. [CrossRef]

16. Nakajima, S.; Takeuchi, H.; Fervaha, G.; Plitman, E.; Chung, J.K.; Caravaggio, F.; Iwata, Y.; Mihashi, Y.; Gerretsen, P.; Remington, G.; et al. Comparative efficacy between clozapine and other atypical antipsychotics on depressive symptoms in patients with schizophrenia: Analysis of the CATIE phase 2E data. *Schizophr. Res.* **2015**, *161*, 429–433. [CrossRef]

17. Wykes, T.; Haro, J.M.; Belli, S.R.; Obradors-Tarragó, C.; Arango, C.; Ayuso-Mateos, J.L.; Bitter, I.; Brunn, M.; Chevreul, K.; Demotes-Mainard, J.; et al. Mental health research priorities for Europe. *Lancet Psychiatry* **2015**, *2*, 1036–1042. [CrossRef]

18. Cipriani, A.; Furukawa, T.A.; Salanti, G.; Chaimani, A.; Atkinson, L.Z.; Ogawa, Y.; Leucht, S.; Ruhe, H.G.; Turner, E.H.; Higgins, J.P.T.; et al. Comparative efficacy and acceptability of 21 antidepressant drugs for the acute treatment of adults with major depressive disorder: A systematic review and network meta-analysis. *Lancet Lond. Engl.* **2018**, *391*, 1357–1366. [CrossRef]

19. Zhu, X.; Han, Y.; Du, J.; Liu, R.; Jin, K.; Yi, W. Microbiota-gut-brain axis and the central nervous system. *Oncotarget* **2017**, *8*, 53829–53838. [CrossRef]

20. Fond, G.; Chevalier, G.; Eberl, G.; Leboyer, M. The potential role of microbiota in major psychiatric disorders: Mechanisms, preclinical data, gastro-intestinal comorbidities and therapeutic options. *Presse Med. Paris Fr. 1983* **2016**, *45*, 7–19.

21. Campos, A.C.; Rocha, N.P.; Nicoli, J.R.; Vieira, L.Q.; Teixeira, M.M.; Teixeira, A.L. Absence of gut microbiota influences lipopolysaccharide-induced behavioral changes in mice. *Behav. Brain Res.* **2016**, *312*, 186–194. [CrossRef]

22. Severance, E.G.; Prandovszky, E.; Castiglione, J.; Yolken, R.H. Gastroenterology issues in schizophrenia: Why the gut matters. *Curr. Psychiatry Rep.* **2015**, *17*, 27. [CrossRef] [PubMed]

23. Severance, E.G.; Gressitt, K.L.; Stallings, C.R.; Origoni, A.E.; Khushalani, S.; Leweke, F.M.; Dickerson, F.B.; Yolken, R.H. Discordant patterns of bacterial translocation markers and implications for innate immune imbalances in schizophrenia. *Schizophr. Res.* **2013**, *148*, 130–137. [CrossRef] [PubMed]

24. Fond, G.; Lançon, C.; Auquier, P.; Boyer, L. C-reactive protein as a peripheral biomarker in schizophrenia. An updated systematic review. *Front. Psychiatry* **2018**, *9*, 392. [CrossRef] [PubMed]

25. Rowland, L.M.; Demyanovich, H.K.; Wijtenburg, S.A.; Eaton, W.W.; Rodriguez, K.; Gaston, F.; Cihakova, D.; Talor, M.V.; Liu, F.; McMahon, R.R.; et al. Antigliadin antibodies (AGA IgG) are related to neurochemistry in schizophrenia. *Front. Psychiatry* **2017**, *8*, 104. [CrossRef]

26. Rook, G.A.W.; Raison, C.L.; Lowry, C.A. Microbiota, immunoregulatory old friends and psychiatric disorders. *Adv. Exp. Med. Biol.* **2014**, *817*, 319–356.

27. Rodrigues-Amorim, D.; Rivera-Baltanás, T.; Regueiro, B.; Spuch, C.; de Las Heras, M.E.; Vázquez-Noguerol Méndez, R.; Nieto-Araujo, M.; Barreiro-Villar, C.; Olivares, J.M.; Agís-Balboa, R.C. The role of the gut microbiota in schizophrenia: Current and future perspectives. *World J. Biol. Psychiatry Off. J. World Fed. Soc. Biol. Psychiatry* **2018**, *19*, 571–585. [CrossRef]

28. Schwarz, E.; Maukonen, J.; Hyytiäinen, T.; Kieseppä, T.; Orešič, M.; Sabunciyan, S.; Mantere, O.; Saarela, M.; Yolken, R.; Suvisaari, J. Analysis of microbiota in first episode psychosis identifies preliminary associations with symptom severity and treatment response. *Schizophr. Res.* **2018**, *192*, 398–403. [CrossRef]

29. Shen, Y.; Xu, J.; Li, Z.; Huang, Y.; Yuan, Y.; Wang, J.; Zhang, M.; Hu, S.; Liang, Y. Analysis of gut microbiota diversity and auxiliary diagnosis as a biomarker in patients with schizophrenia: A cross-sectional study. *Schizophr. Res.* **2018**, *197*, 470–477. [CrossRef]

30. Godin, O.; Leboyer, M.; Gaman, A.; Aouizerate, B.; Berna, F.; Brunel, L.; Capdevielle, D.; Chereau, I.; Dorey, J.M.; Dubertret, C.; et al. Metabolic syndrome, abdominal obesity and hyperuricemia in schizophrenia: Results from the FACE-SZ cohort. *Schizophr. Res.* **2015**, *168*, 388–394. [CrossRef]

31. Fond, G.; Godin, O.; Boyer, L.; Berna, F.; Andrianarisoa, M.; Coulon, N.; Brunel, L.; Bulzacka, E.; Aouizerate, B.; Capdevielle, D.; et al. Chronic low-grade peripheral inflammation is associated with ultra resistant schizophrenia. Results from the FACE-SZ cohort. *Eur. Arch. Psychiatry Clin. Neurosci.* **2018**, *269*, 985–992. [CrossRef]

32. Fond, G.; Resseguier, N.; Schürhoff, F.; Godin, O.; Andrianarisoa, M.; Brunel, L.; Bulzacka, E.; Aouizerate, B.; Berna, F.; Capdevielle, D.; et al. Relationships between low-grade peripheral inflammation and psychotropic drugs in schizophrenia: Results from the national FACE-SZ cohort. *Eur. Arch. Psychiatry Clin. Neurosci.* **2017**, *268*, 541–553. [CrossRef] [PubMed]

33. Fond, G.; Berna, F.; Andrianarisoa, M.; Godin, O.; Leboyer, M.; Brunel, L.; Aouizerate, B.; Capdevielle, D.; Chereau, I.; D'Amato, T.; et al. Chronic low-grade peripheral inflammation is associated with severe nicotine dependence in schizophrenia: Results from the national multicentric FACE-SZ cohort. *Eur. Arch. Psychiatry Clin. Neurosci.* **2017**, *267*, 465–472. [CrossRef] [PubMed]

34. Fond, G.; Godin, O.; Brunel, L.; Aouizerate, B.; Berna, F.; Bulzacka, E.; Capdevielle, D.; Chereau, I.; Dorey, J.M.; Dubertret, C.; et al. Peripheral sub-inflammation is associated with antidepressant consumption in schizophrenia. Results from the multi-center FACE-SZ data set. *J. Affect. Disord.* **2016**, *191*, 209–215. [CrossRef] [PubMed]

35. Faugere, M.; Micoulaud-Franchi, J.-A.; Faget-Agius, C.; Lançon, C.; Cermolacce, M.; Richieri, R. High C-reactive protein levels are associated with depressive symptoms in schizophrenia. *J. Affect. Disord.* **2018**, *225*, 671–675. [CrossRef] [PubMed]

36. Moher, D.; Liberati, A.; Tetzlaff, J.; Altman, D.G. PRISMA Group Preferred reporting items for systematic reviews and meta-analyses: The PRISMA statement. *Br. Med. J.* **2009**, *339*, b2535. [CrossRef] [PubMed]

37. Fond, G.; Loundou, A.; Hamdani, N.; Boukouaci, W.; Dargel, A.; Oliveira, J.; Roger, M.; Tamouza, R.; Leboyer, M.; Boyer, L. Anxiety and depression comorbidities in irritable bowel syndrome (IBS): A systematic review and meta-analysis. *Eur. Arch. Psychiatry Clin. Neurosci.* **2014**, *264*, 651–660. [CrossRef] [PubMed]

38. Peter, J.; Fournier, C.; Durdevic, M.; Knoblich, L.; Keip, B.; Dejaco, C.; Trauner, M.; Moser, G. A Microbial signature of psychological distress in irritable bowel syndrome. *Psychosom. Med.* **2018**, *80*, 698–709. [CrossRef]

39. Kelly, J.R.; Borre, Y.; O' Brien, C.; Patterson, E.; El Aidy, S.; Deane, J.; Kennedy, P.J.; Beers, S.; Scott, K.; Moloney, G.; et al. Transferring the blues: Depression-associated gut microbiota induces neurobehavioural changes in the rat. *J. Psychiatr. Res.* **2016**, *82*, 109–118. [CrossRef]

40. Naseribafrouei, A.; Hestad, K.; Avershina, E.; Sekelja, M.; Linløkken, A.; Wilson, R.; Rudi, K. Correlation between the human fecal microbiota and depression. *Neurogastroenterol. Motil. Off. J. Eur. Gastrointest. Motil. Soc.* **2014**, *26*, 1155–1162. [CrossRef]

41. Kleiman, S.C.; Watson, H.J.; Bulik-Sullivan, E.C.; Huh, E.Y.; Tarantino, L.M.; Bulik, C.M.; Carroll, I.M. The intestinal microbiota in acute anorexia nervosa and during renourishment: Relationship to depression, anxiety, and eating disorder psychopathology. *Psychosom. Med.* **2015**, *77*, 969–981. [CrossRef]

42. Liu, Y.; Zhang, L.; Wang, X.; Wang, Z.; Zhang, J.; Jiang, R.; Wang, X.; Wang, K.; Liu, Z.; Xia, Z.; et al. Similar fecal microbiota signatures in patients with diarrhea-predominant irritable bowel syndrome and patients with depression. *Clin. Gastroenterol. Hepatol. Off. Clin. Pract. J. Am. Gastroenterol. Assoc.* **2016**, *14*, 1602–1611. [CrossRef] [PubMed]

43. Jiang, H.; Ling, Z.; Zhang, Y.; Mao, H.; Ma, Z.; Yin, Y.; Wang, W.; Tang, W.; Tan, Z.; Shi, J.; et al. Altered fecal microbiota composition in patients with major depressive disorder. *Brain. Behav. Immun.* **2015**, *48*, 186–194. [CrossRef] [PubMed]

44. Chen, J.-J.; Zheng, P.; Liu, Y.-Y.; Zhong, X.-G.; Wang, H.-Y.; Guo, Y.-J.; Xie, P. Sex differences in gut microbiota in patients with major depressive disorder. *Neuropsychiatr. Dis. Treat.* **2018**, *14*, 647–655. [CrossRef] [PubMed]

45. Chen, Z.; Li, J.; Gui, S.; Zhou, C.; Chen, J.; Yang, C.; Hu, Z.; Wang, H.; Zhong, X.; Zeng, L.; et al. Comparative metaproteomics analysis shows altered fecal microbiota signatures in patients with major depressive disorder. *Neuroreport* **2018**, *29*, 417–425. [CrossRef] [PubMed]

46. Mason, B.L.; Li, Q.; Minhajuddin, A.; Czysz, A.H.; Coughlin, L.A.; Hussain, S.K.; Koh, A.Y.; Trivedi, M.H. Reduced anti-inflammatory gut microbiota are associated with depression and anhedonia. *J. Affect. Disord.* **2020**, *266*, 394–401. [CrossRef] [PubMed]

47. Madan, A.; Thompson, D.; Fowler, J.C.; Ajami, N.J.; Salas, R.; Frueh, B.C.; Bradshaw, M.R.; Weinstein, B.L.; Oldham, J.M.; Petrosino, J.F. The gut microbiota is associated with psychiatric symptom severity and treatment outcome among individuals with serious mental illness. *J. Affect. Disord.* **2020**, *264*, 98–106. [CrossRef]

48. Lin, P.; Ding, B.; Feng, C.; Yin, S.; Zhang, T.; Qi, X.; Lv, H.; Guo, X.; Dong, K.; Zhu, Y.; et al. Prevotella and Klebsiella proportions in fecal microbial communities are potential characteristic parameters for patients with major depressive disorder. *J. Affect. Disord.* **2017**, *207*, 300–304. [CrossRef]

49. Ng, Q.X.; Soh, A.Y.S.; Venkatanarayanan, N.; Ho, C.Y.X.; Lim, D.Y.; Yeo, W.-S. A systematic review of the effect of probiotic supplementation on schizophrenia symptoms. *Neuropsychobiology* **2019**, *78*, 1–6. [CrossRef]

50. Kiecolt-Glaser, J.K.; Wilson, S.J.; Bailey, M.L.; Andridge, R.; Peng, J.; Jaremka, L.M.; Fagundes, C.P.; Malarkey, W.B.; Laskowski, B.; Belury, M.A. Marital distress, depression, and a leaky gut: Translocation of bacterial endotoxin as a pathway to inflammation. *Psychoneuroendocrinology* **2018**, *98*, 52–60. [CrossRef]

51. Liu, R.T.; Walsh, R.F.L.; Sheehan, A.E. Prebiotics and probiotics for depression and anxiety: A systematic review and meta-analysis of controlled clinical trials. *Neurosci. Biobehav. Rev.* **2019**, *102*, 13–23. [CrossRef]

52. Lagier, J.-C.; Raoult, D. Fecal microbiota transplantation: Indications and perspectives. *Med. Sci. M/S* **2016**, *32*, 991–997.

53. Lagier, J.-C.; Million, M.; Raoult, D. Bouillabaisse or fish soup: The Limitations of meta-analysis confronted to the inconsistency of fecal microbiota transplantation studies. *Clin. Infect. Dis. Off. Publ. Infect. Dis. Soc. Am.* **2019**. [CrossRef] [PubMed]

54. Kump, P.K.; Krause, R.; Allerberger, F.; Högenauer, C. Faecal microbiota transplantation–the Austrian approach. *Clin. Microbiol. Infect. Off. Publ. Eur. Soc. Clin. Microbiol. Infect. Dis.* **2014**, *20*, 1106–1111. [CrossRef] [PubMed]

55. Cui, B.; Feng, Q.; Wang, H.; Wang, M.; Peng, Z.; Li, P.; Huang, G.; Liu, Z.; Wu, P.; Fan, Z.; et al. Fecal microbiota transplantation through mid-gut for refractory Crohn's disease: Safety, feasibility, and efficacy trial results. *J. Gastroenterol. Hepatol.* **2015**, *30*, 51–58. [CrossRef]

56. Hocquart, M.; Lagier, J.-C.; Cassir, N.; Saidani, N.; Eldin, C.; Kerbaj, J.; Delord, M.; Valles, C.; Brouqui, P.; Raoult, D.; et al. Early fecal microbiota transplantation improves survival in severe clostridium difficile infections. *Clin. Infect. Dis. Off. Publ. Infect. Dis. Soc. Am.* **2018**, *66*, 645–650. [CrossRef]

57. Van Nood, E.; Vrieze, A.; Nieuwdorp, M.; Fuentes, S.; Zoetendal, E.G.; de Vos, W.M.; Visser, C.E.; Kuijper, E.J.; Bartelsman, J.F.W.M.; Tijssen, J.G.P.; et al. Duodenal infusion of donor feces for recurrent Clostridium difficile. *N. Engl. J. Med.* **2013**, *368*, 407–415. [CrossRef]

58. Austin, M.; Mellow, M.; Tierney, W.M. Fecal microbiota transplantation in the treatment of Clostridium difficile infections. *Am. J. Med.* **2014**, *127*, 479–483. [CrossRef]

59. Cammarota, G.; Masucci, L.; Ianiro, G.; Bibbò, S.; Dinoi, G.; Costamagna, G.; Sanguinetti, M.; Gasbarrini, A. Randomised clinical trial: Faecal microbiota transplantation by colonoscopy vs. vancomycin for the treatment of recurrent Clostridium difficile infection. *Aliment. Pharmacol. Ther.* **2015**, *41*, 835–843. [CrossRef]

60. Li, Y.-T.; Cai, H.-F.; Wang, Z.-H.; Xu, J.; Fang, J.-Y. Systematic review with meta-analysis: Long-term outcomes of faecal microbiota transplantation for Clostridium difficile infection. *Aliment. Pharmacol. Ther.* **2016**, *43*, 445–457. [CrossRef]

61. Paramsothy, S.; Kamm, M.A.; Kaakoush, N.O.; Walsh, A.J.; van den Bogaerde, J.; Samuel, D.; Leong, R.W.L.; Connor, S.; Ng, W.; Paramsothy, R.; et al. Multidonor intensive faecal microbiota transplantation for active ulcerative colitis: A randomised placebo-controlled trial. *Lancet* **2017**, *389*, 1218–1228. [CrossRef]

62. Costello, S.P.; Hughes, P.A.; Waters, O.; Bryant, R.V.; Vincent, A.D.; Blatchford, P.; Katsikeros, R.; Makanyanga, J.; Campaniello, M.A.; Mavrangelos, C.; et al. Effect of fecal microbiota transplantation on 8-week remission in patients with ulcerative colitis: A randomized clinical trial. *JAMA* **2019**, *321*, 156–164. [CrossRef] [PubMed]

63. Johnsen, P.H.; Hilpüsch, F.; Cavanagh, J.P.; Leikanger, I.S.; Kolstad, C.; Valle, P.C.; Goll, R. Faecal microbiota transplantation versus placebo for moderate-to-severe irritable bowel syndrome: A double-blind, randomised, placebo-controlled, parallel-group, single-centre trial. *Lancet Gastroenterol. Hepatol.* **2018**, *3*, 17–24. [CrossRef]

64. Wang, S.; Xu, M.; Wang, W.; Cao, X.; Piao, M.; Khan, S.; Yan, F.; Cao, H.; Wang, B. Systematic review: Adverse events of fecal microbiota transplantation. *PLoS ONE* **2016**, *11*, e0161174. [CrossRef] [PubMed]

65. Flint, H.J. Obesity and the gut microbiota. *J. Clin. Gastroenterol.* **2011**, *45*, S128–S132. [CrossRef] [PubMed]

66. Rao, K.; Young, V.B.; Malani, P.N. Capsules for fecal microbiota transplantation in recurrent clostridium difficile Infection: The new way forward or a tough pill to swallow? *JAMA* **2017**, *318*, 1979–1980. [CrossRef]

67. Kao, D.; Roach, B.; Silva, M.; Beck, P.; Rioux, K.; Kaplan, G.G.; Chang, H.-J.; Coward, S.; Goodman, K.J.; Xu, H.; et al. Effect of oral capsule- vs colonoscopy-delivered fecal microbiota transplantation on recurrent clostridium difficile infection: A randomized clinical trial. *JAMA* **2017**, *318*, 1985–1993. [CrossRef]

68. Staley, C.; Hamilton, M.J.; Vaughn, B.P.; Graiziger, C.T.; Newman, K.M.; Kabage, A.J.; Sadowsky, M.J.; Khoruts, A. Successful resolution of recurrent clostridium difficile infection using freeze-dried, encapsulated fecal microbiota; pragmatic cohort study. *Am. J. Gastroenterol.* **2017**, *112*, 940–947. [CrossRef]

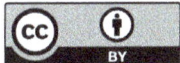

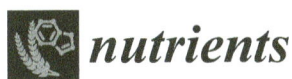

Review

The Association between Energy Balance-Related Behavior and Burn-Out in Adults: A Systematic Review

Yanni Verhavert [1,*], Kristine De Martelaer [1,2], Elke Van Hoof [3], Eline Van Der Linden [1], Evert Zinzen [1] and Tom Deliens [1]

[1] Department of Movement and Sport Sciences, Vrije Universiteit Brussel, Pleinlaan 2, 1050 Brussels, Belgium; kdmartel@vub.be (K.D.M.); eline.van.der.linden@vub.be (E.V.D.L.); evert.zinzen@vub.be (E.Z.); tom.deliens@vub.be (T.D.)
[2] Faculty of Social and Behavioral Sciences, Utrecht University, Heidelberglaan 1, 3584 CS Utrecht, The Netherlands
[3] Department of Psychology, Vrije Universiteit Brussel, Pleinlaan 2, 1050 Brussels, Belgium; elke.van.hoof@vub.be
*   Correspondence: yanni.verhavert@vub.be

Received: 28 November 2019; Accepted: 31 January 2020; Published: 2 February 2020

Abstract: Although it is believed that physical activity, sedentary, and dietary behavior (i.e., energy balance-related behavior) may decrease the risk of burn-out, the association between both is currently not well understood. Therefore, the aim of this systematic review was to synthesize studies investigating the relationship between energy balance-related behavior and burn-out risk. A systematic literature search was conducted in four databases, resulting in 25 included studies (ten experimental and 15 observational studies). Nine out of ten experimental studies showed that exercise programs were effective in reducing burn-out risk. Fourteen out of fifteen observational studies found a negative association between physical activity and burn-out risk, whereas one study did not find a relation. Two of the 15 observational studies also showed that being more sedentary was associated with a higher burn-out risk, and two other studies found that a healthier diet was related to a lower burn-out risk. No experimental studies were found for the latter two behaviors. It can be concluded that physical activity may be effective in reducing burn-out risk. The few observational studies linking sedentary and dietary behavior with burn-out risk suggest that being more sedentary and eating less healthy are each associated with higher burn-out risk. More high-quality research is needed to unravel the causal relationship between these two behaviors and burn-out risk.

Keywords: mental health; emotional exhaustion; cynicism; professional efficacy; physical activity; sedentary behavior; dietary behavior

1. Introduction

Over recent decades, the prevalence—but also the recognition—of burn-out has increased enormously [1,2]. Burn-out often leads to absenteeism and presenteeism at work [3–5], and so it is an increasing concern in today's workplaces [6]. In the European Union, work-related stress costs EUR 25.4 billion annually, whereas globally, burn-out and stress cost more than USD 300 billion every year [7,8].

Burn-out can be defined as a "prolonged response to chronic emotional and interpersonal stressors on the job, determined by three dimensions: emotional exhaustion, cynicism or depersonalization, and professional (in)efficacy or personal accomplishment" [9]. People experiencing burn-out are mainly mentioning feelings of mental and physical exhaustion, low mood and lack of energy, and therefore emotional exhaustion is seen as the key component of burn-out [1,9,10]. To have better insight into the relationships people have with their job, it is also important to include the other two dimensions. Cynicism refers to the cognitive distance burned out people are taking from their job, and professional (in)efficacy refers to the feeling of being incompetent at work [9,11].

To reduce the high—and increasing—incidence and prevalence of burn-out, effective interventions are needed. In a systematic review by Awa et al. [12], it was concluded that a lot of interventions, such as relaxation training and task restructuring at work, are effective, but after several months the positive effects are diminished. This shows the need to develop interventions that are effective in the long term. It has been argued that energy balance-related behavior—including physical activity, sedentary and dietary behavior—may play an important role in preventing and/or curing burn-out. Although physical (in)activity and diet have been associated with mental health, depression and anxiety [13–15], their link with burn-out is unclear. There are several reasons why energy balance-related behavior may be effective to reduce and prevent burn-out.

Physical activity is defined as "any bodily movement produced by skeletal muscles and which requires energy expenditure" [16]. The benefits of physical activity and exercise are enormous. Besides the well-known cardiovascular adaptations, they can increase cerebral blood flow, upregulate neurotrophic factors (e.g., brain-derived neurotrophic factor (BDNF)), support cognitive function and improve executive functions (e.g., planning and sequencing) [17–19]. Furthermore, physical activity can facilitate taking psychological distance from work, which reduces job stress and increases job performance [20,21]. As people with burn-out have decreased BDNF-levels, increased job stress, and decreased cognitive function, the abovementioned benefits of physical activity may reduce or even prevent burn-out [22–24]. In a systematic review by Naczenski et al. [1], which included ten studies, it was concluded that physical activity may be effective in reducing burn-out levels, showing a possible causal relationship between both. On the other hand, a systematic review and meta-analysis by Ochentel et al. [6] did not find clear (statistical) evidence that exercise therapy is effective in reducing burn-out levels. It should be said, though, that the majority of the included studies in the meta-analysis reported significant differences between the intervention and control groups. Moreover, only four studies were meta-analyzed, making it difficult to make reliable statistical statements.

Sedentary behavior is defined as "any waking behavior characterized by an energy expenditure ≤ 1.5 METs (Metabolic Equivalent of Task) while in a sitting, reclining or lying posture" [25]. Sedentary behavior is associated with physical (in)activity [26], but there is still a clear distinction between both [27,28]. A systematic review by Rezende et al. [29] concluded that sedentary behavior may be a determinant of health, independently of physical activity. In addition, van der Ploeg et al. [27] indicated that sedentary behavior and physical (in)activity should be targeted at the same time in public health strategies, while the two earlier mentioned systematic reviews [1,6], only included studies assessing the link between physical activity and burn-out, without taking sedentary behavior into account. It has been suggested that sedentary behavior may influence mental performance and mental health. Watching television, for example, is associated with decreased executive functioning and decreased cognitive performance [30,31]. Furthermore, Engeroff et al. [32] found that BDNF-levels are negatively associated with sedentary behavior. In a systematic review by Teychenne et al. [33] it was suggested that sedentary behavior is associated with a higher risk of depression, while an experimental study demonstrated that increased sedentary time may result in decreased mood [34].

Dietary behavior is another component of energy balance-related behavior and includes aspects such as dietary intake, diet quality and dietary patterns. Diet may also play a role in reducing and preventing burn-out, as it exerts a certain influence on neurotransmitters and neurotransmission. Research showed that the function and levels of neurotransmitters are different in people with burn-out [35,36]. Tops et al. [35] found that people experiencing burn-out are showing a low serotonergic and a low dopaminergic function. Furthermore, low exhaustion is associated with higher neurotransmitter levels, such as norepinephrine, dopamine and acetylcholine, compared to people with moderate exhaustion [36]. It should be mentioned that, in the latter study, a comparison with people experiencing high exhaustion could not be made due to the lack of highly exhausted people. Previous research has already demonstrated the mediating role of neurotransmission in the relationship between diet and mental health. For example, the administration of tryptophan increases brain serotonin synthesis, which, in turn, influences serotonin-dependent brain functions such as mood [37]. Tryptophan can be found in foods such as poultry, milk and some seeds. Likewise, the administration of tyrosine increases the production and release of dopamine and norepinephrine [37], which was found to be diminished in exhausted people. Tryptophan can be found in foods such as poultry, milk and some seeds. Likewise, the administration of tyrosine increases the production and release of dopamine and norepinephrine [37], which was found to be diminished in exhausted people. An increased production and release of this amino acid can be useful in enhancing performance during highly stressful situations. Tyrosine can be found in foods such as dairy, meat and fish. Secondly, studies showed that glucose administration and dietary carbohydrates enhance cognitive performance [38–40], while Chung et al. [41] suggested that also a mixed-grain diet can be beneficial for cognitive performance. This latter study also found beneficial effects of mixed-grain diet on plasma BDNF levels, which are decreased in people with burn-out. Lastly, omega-3-supplementation is associated with mood state, which results in an increase in feelings of vigor and a decrease in feelings of anger, anxiety, fatigue, depression and confusion [42]. The abovementioned physiological mechanisms hypothesize the preventative and healing functions of energy balance-related behavior towards burn-out.

It is clear that—given the rise in incidence and prevalence of burn-out—effective interventions are urgently needed. Improving energy balance-related behavior may be a promising strategy to counter burn-out. Although two recent (contradicting) systematic reviews [1,6] on the single association between physical activity and burn-out have been published, to date, no overview of studies investigating the relationship between energy balance-related behavior from a holistic point of view (including physical activity, sedentary and dietary behavior) and burn-out is available. Therefore, the aim of the present systematic review is to synthesize studies investigating the association between energy balance-related behavior and burn-out.

2. Materials and Methods

This review is registered in PROSPERO with registration number: CRD42019124458.

2.1. PICO Statement

The present systematic review investigates the association between energy balance-related behavior (i.e., physical activity, sedentary and dietary behavior) (=exposure or intervention) and burn-out (=outcome) in adults (=population).

2.2. Databases and Key Words

Following the PRISMA guidelines for conducting systematic reviews [43], a search was conducted in PubMed, Web of Science, PsycINFO and Embase using the following search terms: "energy balance-related behavior", "energy balance", "energy expenditure", "physical (in)activity", "physically (in)active", "exercise", "training", "sport", "moving", "work-out", "leisure (time) activity", "walking", "biking", "(in)active lifestyle", "lifestyle (related) activity", "household activity", "housework", "gardening", "active transport", "transportation", "sedentary", "sitting", "lying down", "diet", "food", "eating", "nutrition", "caloric intake", "energy intake", "burn-out", "affective disorder", "adaptive disorder", "common mental disorder", "psychological discomfort", "psychological stress", "psychological health", "psychological illness", "psychological fatigue", "job stress", "toxic stress", "chronic stress", "work stress", "occupational stress", "occupational health", "exhaustion", "mental fatigue", "mental illness"; "mental disorder", "well-being", "emotional burden", "depersonalisation", "personal accomplishment", "cynicism", "inefficacy". The PICO/PECO method [44] was used to structure and combine key words using Boolean terms. Wildcards were used for plural, other spelling and to cover British and American English equivalents.

2.3. Eligibility Criteria

Results were limited to original English-language articles published in full-text format in peer reviewed journals until January 2019, assessing the direct relationship between energy balance-related behavior (i.e., physical activity, sedentary and dietary behavior) and burn-out or one or more of its components (i.e., emotional exhaustion, cynicism and inefficacy) in working adults between 18 and 65 years old. Meta-analyses, systematic reviews, methodological papers, congress proceedings, meeting abstracts and case studies were excluded from the search. Studies were also excluded when investigating other affective disorders than burn-out (such as depression, bipolar disorders and anxiety disorders), investigating the influence of an intervention including more than only physical activity (such a mediation exercises, workshops, etc.) on burn-out levels, including non-working adults such as people in prison, students, athletes, etc., investigating the association between burn-out and disordered eating behaviors (such as emotional eating, uncontrolled eating, etc.), or investigating the association between burn-out and alcohol.

2.4. Selection of Studies

After completing the search in each database, all references were imported into EndNote (=bibliographic software program) and then exported to Rayyan (=bibliographic software program designed to facilitate systematic reference selection), in which the study selection was conducted. The study selection included the screening of titles, abstract and full-texts and conducting a forward and backward search. The search and study selection were conducted in January 2019 by two researchers independently from each other (YV and EVDL). Any doubts or disagreements between the two researchers were discussed with a third researcher (TD). The followed methodology was reviewed and approved by the head of the university library (KA). When important information in the articles was missing, authors were contacted via e-mail.

2.5. Quality Assessment

The 'Standard quality assessment criteria for evaluating primary research papers from a variety of fields' [45] was used to assess the methodological quality of the included studies. The checklist consists of 14 items which were given a certain score depending on whether or not the specific criterion was met ("no" = 0, "partial" = 1, "yes" = 2). Depending on the study design, some items were not applicable and were therefore scored as 'not applicable (N/A)' and excluded from the calculation of the total score. The total sum was calculated by summing the total number of "yes" multiplied by 2 and the total number of "partials" multiplied by 1. The total possible sum was calculated as follows: 28 − (number of 'N/A' × 2). Lastly, the summary score was calculated by dividing the total sum by the total possible sum.

3. Results

In total, 18,536 articles were found. When removing all duplicates, 4907 articles remained. Titles and abstracts were screened for eligibility. Of the 109 remaining articles, sixteen studies met the inclusion criteria. In addition, a forward and backward search was performed through which we identified six more studies. Another two articles were included after screening the reference lists of two previously published systematic reviews investigating the association between physical activity and burn-out [1,6]. One more article was obtained through hand search [46]. So, in total, 25 articles were included in the final synthesis. The flow chart of the search process is displayed in Figure 1.

Nutrients **2020**, *12*, 397

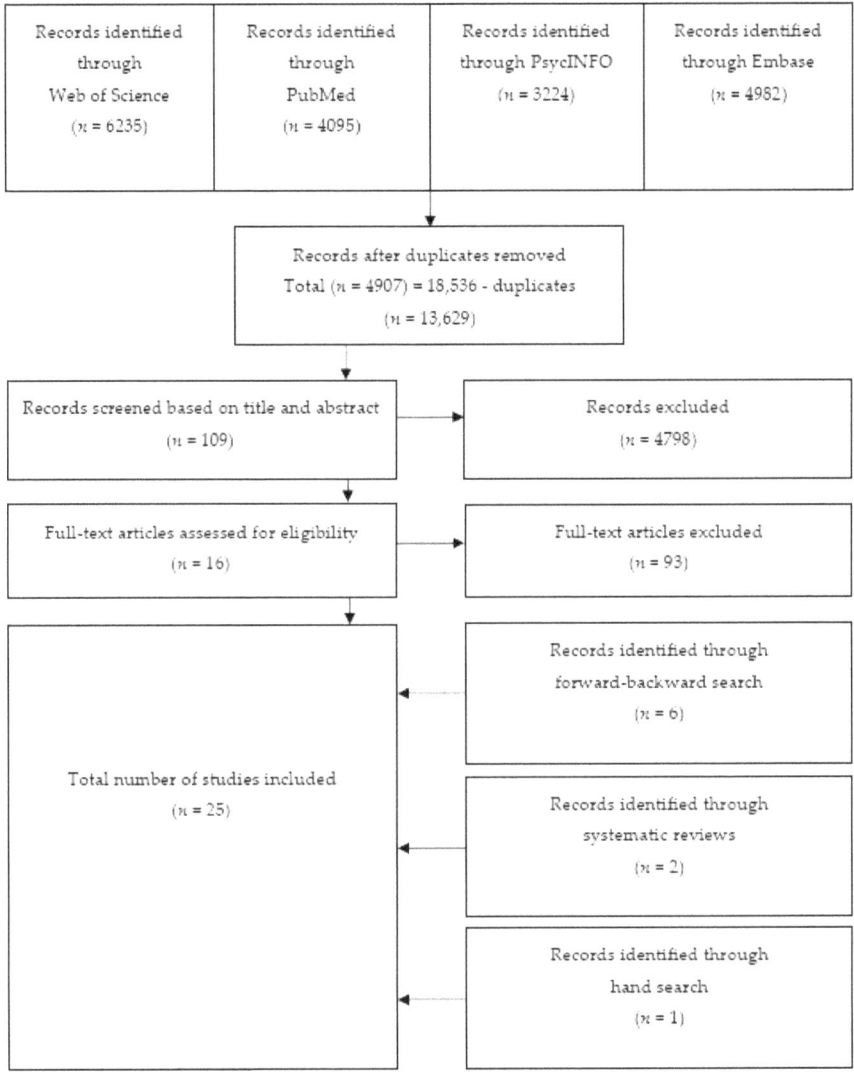

Figure 1. Flow chart of the systematic search.

The 25 included studies consisted of ten experimental and 15 observational studies. The experimental studies included five randomized controlled trials (RCTs), one randomized clinical trial, one quasi experimental and three pre-experimental studies. An overview of the included experimental studies is presented in Table 1. The observational studies included six longitudinal and nine cross-sectional studies. An overview of the included observational studies is presented in Table 2.

Table 1. Overview of the included experimental studies.

Author (year) and Country	Design	Participants and Setting	Intervention	Timing of Measurements	Outcome Measure and Measurement Tool	Conclusion
			Physical activity			
De Vries et al. [47] The Netherlands	RCT	96 employees with high levels of work-related fatigue: - 19 men, 77 women - Mean age: 45.2 ± 1.6 years	Exercise intervention: 1 h low-intensity running sessions three times a week for 6 consecutive weeks. Wait-list control: participants were offered the opportunity to follow the intervention after the 6 weeks training of the IG.	IG: pre-intervention and post-intervention, 6 and 12 weeks after intervention period. CG: pre-intervention and post-intervention.	Work-related fatigue: five-item 'exhaustion'-subscale of the Dutch version of the MBI.	Exercise is effective to reduce emotional exhaustion (T0-T1: cohen's $d = -0.62$; -21.6%; $p = 0.04$). Small improvements in emotional exhaustion 6 weeks after the end of the intervention. These were maintained at 12 weeks (T0-T2: cohen's $d = -1.03$; -33.8%; $p < 0.01$; T0-T3: cohen's $d = -1.06$; -32.6% $p < 0.01$; T1-T2: cohen's $d = -0.3$, -15.6%, $p < 0.05$). No significant difference between T1 and T3 and between T2 and T3.
Dreyer et al. [48] New Zealand	RCT	81 staff members at a college: - 25 men, 56 women - Mean age: 42.1 years	The exercise intervention lasted for 10 weeks (4–5 days per week). The exercise intervention: a combination of aerobic exercise (cycling, stair climber, treadmill running) and resistance exercise. Aerobic exercise: participants started at 40–50% of age-adjusted maximum heart rate with 40-min sessions for the first 2 weeks, followed by 50–60% with 30-min sessions during the next 3 weeks, and 70% or higher with 20-min sessions for the last 4 weeks. Resistance exercise: 4–5 sets of 4 exercises with a 30-second recovery interval between sets. The entire circuit had to be completed within 40 min. CG: no intervention.	Pre, post (week immediately after the intervention).	Emotional exhaustion: Psychological Burn-out Questionnaire.	Emotional exhaustion improved significantly after the 10-week exercise intervention (-10%).

Table 1. *Cont.*

Author (year) and Country	Design	Participants and Setting	Intervention	Timing of Measurements	Outcome Measure and Measurement Tool	Conclusion
Eskilsson et al. [49] Sweden	RCT	56 patients with exhaustion disorder. All patients were on sick leave: - 4 men, 52 women - Mean age: 41.8 ± 8.2 years	Multimodal rehabilitation program containing components of group-based or individual cognitive behavioral therapy, physical activities and work training coordinated by an interdisciplinary team. 12-week intervention: Aerobic training was performed as group indoor cycling (spinning), 40 min, 3 times per week. Intensity: 70–85% of their maximum age-adjusted heart rate. CG: Multimodal rehabilitation program with no additional training.	Baseline, week 12, week 24.	Burn-out: SMBQ.	No additional improvement in burn-out in the aerobic group compared to controls. Levels of burn-out improved equally in both groups (aerobic training group: T1-T2: −17.5%, no *p*-value mentioned).
Freitas et al. [50] Brazil	Pre-experiment	21 nursing professionals (from the Barretos Cancer Hospital): - 1 man, 20 women - Mean age: 37.4 ± 9.1 years - employed for 1 year or more	The compensatory workplace PA was conducted 5 days/week, lasting 10 min, during 3 consecutive months. No CG.	Pre, post	Burn-out: MBI	No significant difference in the three dimensions of burn-out between pre- and post-intervention.
Gerber et al. [51] Swiss	Pre-experiment	Employees with high levels of work-related burn-out: - 12 men - Mean age: 45.8 ± 6.8 years	12-week exercise-training program, 2–3 times a week, 60 min: aerobic exercise program based on the exercise prescription guidelines of the American College of Sports Medicine. 60–75% of their maximum heart rate. No CG.	Pre, post (3 days after the 12-week intervention).	Burn-out: German version of the MBI.	Burn-out symptoms were significantly reduced after the 12-week aerobic exercise program. Emotional exhaustion and depersonalization were reduced. No significant changes were found for personal accomplishment (Emotional exhaustion: T1-T2: cohen's d = 1.84; −33.4%; *p* < 0.001; depersonalization: T1-T2: cohen's d = 1.35; −33.5%; *p* < 0.001; personal accomplishment: T1-T2: no significant difference).

Table 1. *Cont.*

Author (year) and Country	Design	Participants and Setting	Intervention	Timing of Measurements	Outcome Measure and Measurement Tool	Conclusion
Heiden et al. [52] Sweden	RCT	75 patients being on sick leave for at least 50% of the time for 1 month to 2 years due to stress-related illnesses: - 15 men, 60 women - Mean age: 44.0 ± 9.0 years	PA programme: 2 exercise sessions per week for 10 weeks. Session 1: a rehabilitation program with low-intensity exercises in a warm water pool. Session 2: the participants chose an exercise (e.g., strength training, swimming, aerobics or walking). During the intervention, each participant kept a diary of their physical exercise. The cognitive behavioral training programme focused on cognitive restructuring to improve self-care behavior and social support. CG: usual care provided by the Swedish social insurance system during the course of the study. Participants were promised treatment after the study was completed.	Pre, post, at 6 and at 12 months after the intervention.	Burn-out: SMBQ.	Participants rated lower levels of burn-out after the intervention period (F=10.0; p = 0.002). At the 6-month follow up assessment, patients' ratings of burn-out continued to improve. At 12 months after the intervention, similar results were found. Little difference in the effect of cognitive behavioral training and PA, compared with usual care, was found (PA intervention: pre-post: −12.1%; cognitive behavioral training; pre-post: −12.9%; usual care pre-post: +2.9%, no *p*-values mentioned)
Lindegard et al. [53] Sweden	Pre-experiment	69 patients with exhaustion disorder on sick leave for less than 6 months: - 24 men, 69 women - Mean age: 42.6 ± 1.4 years - Only physically inactive patients at baseline were included.	Multimodel treatment for 12 months and a special focus was placed on PA counselling; an 8-week group stress management program. All patients were given background information on the causes and consequences of chronic stress during a 2-h lecture. They were visiting every 4–6 weeks a physician and the program consisted of a 2 h lecture about stress-related mental disorders and the consequences on the individual and organisational level. The participants were also given comprehensive information of the effects of regular PA on stress-related exhaustion, opportunity to self-select their participation in an 18-week coached group exercise-program. Exercise program: Nordic walking for 1 h and a light strength-training program performed at the clinic once a week. No CG.	Pre, at 6 months, at 12 months, at 18 months.	Burn-out: SMBQ. PA activity: at baseline: with the SGPALS, at follow-up: "How often did you exercise during the last 3 months?" and "How hard did you normally exercise during the last 3 months?" and "How many minutes did you engage in activity?"	Mild and strong compliers reported significantly lower burn-out at the 18-month follow-up than the non-complying group (pre-18 months: non-compliers: −27.7%; mild-compliers: −47.8%; strong compliers: −41.3%; $p < 0.017$).

Table 1. *Cont.*

Author (year) and Country	Design	Participants and Setting	Intervention	Timing of Measurements	Outcome Measure and Measurement Tool	Conclusion
Stenlund et al. [54] Sweden	RCT	82 patients with burn-out: - 14 men, 68 women - Mean age: 44.3 ± 9.1 years	IG: Qigong twice a week (1-h sessions) for 12 weeks. The Qigong program: warm-up movements, basic movements to affect body awareness, balance and coordination, breathing and muscular tension, and relaxation and mindfulness meditation. The IG also took part in basic care at the Stress Clinic. The CG took part in basic care at the Stress Clinic.	Pre, at week 4 and week 8 of the intervention and after the intervention.	Burn-out: SMBQ.	Both groups improved significantly with reduced levels of burn-out. No additional effects of Qigong on recovery in burn-out patients compared to basic care for patients with burn-out (IG: pre-post: -6.9%; $p \le 0.001$; CG: pre-post: -17.4%; $p < 0.001$).
Tsai et al. [55] China	Quasi-experiment	89 banking and insurance workers: - Low intensity group: $n = 30$, 11 men, 19 women, mean age: 34.8 ± 7.0 years - High intensity: $n = 29$, 3 men, 27 women, mean age: 41.0 ± 7.2 years - CG: $n = 29$, 10 men, 19 women, mean age: 33.3 ± 9.4 years.	12-week exercise program: gymnastics (15 min); aerobic exercise (30 min) and stretching (15 min). Low-intensity group: participants were assigned to attend 1 exercise session per week. High-intensity group: participants were assigned to attend 2 exercise sessions per week. Participants planned and carried out exercise regimes on their own.	Pre, post	Work-related burn-out: CBI.	The exercise program improved work-related burn-out. (High-intensity exercise: pre- post: -8.1%; low-intensity exercise: pre-post: -8.2%; no p-values mentioned).
Van Rhenen et al. [56] The Netherlands	Randomised clinical trial	75 employees working in a telecommunications company: - Sex distribution not mentioned. - Age: between 18.0 and 63.0 years	Condition 1: Physical intervention: to provide awareness and introduction of physical and relaxation exercises in daily work activities. The level and intensity of the exercises were modified in such a way that it met the physical capability of each individual. The sessions took place during working hrs. Four sessions, each lasting for 1 h, were given over a period of 8 weeks. Every session consisted of 4 main parts: introduction, warming-up and physical exercise, relaxation exercise and an assignment. Condition 2: Stressed cognitive intervention: to restructure irrational beliefs. Participants were randomly assigned to 1 of the 2 conditions. No CG.	Pre, 10 weeks and 6 months after the training period.	Burn-out: UBOS, the Dutch version of the MBI-General Survey.	Both interventions had a positive effect on exhaustion and cynicism in both the short and long term (physical intervention: exhaustion: pre-post: -10%; $p = 0.04$; cynicism: pre-post: -4%; $p = 0.04$; cognitive intervention: exhaustion: pre-post: -4%; $p = 0.04$; cynicism: pre-post: -9.3%; $p = 0.04$).

Abbreviations: Maslach Burn-out Inventory (MBI), Shirom-Melamed Burn-out Questionnaire (SMBQ), Copenhagen Burn-out Inventory (CBI), Utrechtse Burn-out Schaal (UBOS), Physical Activity (PA) Intervention group (IG), Control group (CG), Randomised Controlled Trial (RCT).

Table 2. Overview of the included observational studies.

Author (year) and Country	Design	Participants and Setting	Outcome Measure and Measurement Tools	Conclusion
		Physical activity		
Ahola et al. [57] Finland	Cross-sectional	3264 participants: - 1645 men, 1619 women - Mean age: 44.5 years	Burn-out: MBI - General Survey. Leisure-time PA: questionnaire. Participants who reported spending at least 4 h of their weekly leisure-time in physical activities = "active", and those who reported spending most of their leisure-time in non-physical activities = "passive".	Burn-out syndrome was related to low PA: OR, 1.21; 95% CI, 1.12–1.30). Exhaustion (OR, 1.23; 95% CI, 1.12–1.32), cynicism (OR, 1.10; 95% CI, 1.01–1.19) and a lack of professional efficacy (OR, 1.13; 95% CI, 1.06–1.22) were associated with low PA levels.
Bernaards et al. [58] The Netherlands	Longitudinal with 4 time points: baseline measurements between 1994 and 1995, and follow-up measurements in 1996, 1997 and 1998.	1747 workers from 34 companies (blue-and white-collar jobs and caring professions) - Sex distribution and age were not mentioned. - Participants had to be employed in their current job for at least 1 year and work at least 24 h per week.	Emotional exhaustion: it was assessed with one of the three subscales from an adapted Dutch version of the MBI. Strenuous PA: "How often within the past four months did you participate in strenuous sports activities or strenuous physical activities that lasted long enough to become sweaty?" The amount of sedentary work: participants reporting sitting during the largest part of the working day = workers with a sedentary job, participants not reporting sitting during the largest part of the working day = worker with a non-sedentary job.	All workers who engaged in strenuous PA at a frequency of one to twice a week were at a significant lower risk of emotional exhaustion than workers who engaged in strenuous PA less than once a month. This association was stronger in workers with a sedentary job. PA at a frequency of once to twice a week was significantly associated with a reduced risk of future emotional exhaustion, this was not the case for PA at a higher frequency. (1–2x per week: non-sedentary job: OR, 0.70; 95% CI, 0.51–0.97; sedentary job: OR, 0.48; 95% CI, 0.30–0.76)
Carson et al. [59] USA	Cross-sectional	189 full-time childcare teachers (African, American, Caucasian-American): - 1 man, 188 women - Mean age: 33.6 ± 12.4 years	Emotional exhaustion: the nine-item emotional exhaustion subscale from the MBI-Educators Survey. Self-reported PA behavior: Habitual Physical Activity Questionnaire. 16 items delineated into 3 distinct indices: work index, sport-related index and leisure-time index.	Work related PA ($r = -0.3$, $p < 0.01$) and leisure-time PA ($r = -0.19$, $p < 0.05$) were negatively correlated with emotional exhaustion.
de Vries et al. [60] The Netherlands	Longitudinal with 2 time points: measurements in 2008 and 2009.	2275 full-time employees: - 75.3% men → mean age: 45.8 ± 10.0 years 24.7% women → mean age: 39.9 ±11.4 years) - The participants primarily worked in the area of business services, public administration, industry, and education (no physically demanding jobs) - Mean working hrs per week: 38.4 ± 3.1 - Mean working days per week: 4.9 ± 0.5	Work-related fatigue: five-item 'exhaustion'-subscale of the Dutch version of the MBI. PA: questionnaire based on international standards for PA: "On how many days a week are you normally physically active during at least 30 min a day during your work and free time together (only count PA that is equally demanding as brisk walking or biking. Activities shorter than 10 min do not count)?"	It was found that an increase in PA is associated with a decrease in work-related fatigue over time ($\beta = -0.05$, $p < 0.05$). Cross-sectionally, work-related fatigue is negatively correlated with PA at T1 and T2 (T1: $r = -0.08$, $p < 0.01$; T2: $r = -0.08$, $p < 0.001$)

Table 2. *Cont.*

Author (year) and Country	Design	Participants and Setting	Outcome Measure and Measurement Tools	Conclusion
Liang et al. [61] Taiwan	Longitudinal	197 full-time employees in five manufacturing industries: - 163 men, 34 women - Age: not mentioned	Burn-out: CBI. Exercise behavior: 5 questions on a 5-point scale: 1 = never and 5 = many times in a week. Example questions: "How many times in a week do you take part in sports that include aerobic exercise (e.g., basketball and running)?" and "How many times in a week do you engage in aerobic exercise for at least 30 min?"	Work-related burn-out was negatively correlated with exercise behavior ($r = -0.22$, $p < 0.01$).
Lindwall et al. [62] Sweden	Longitudinal with 5 time points: baseline, in 2004, in 2006, in 2008 and in 2010.	3717 health care workers: - Sex distribution not mentioned. - Mean age: 46.9 ± 10.0 years - Criteria for inclusion: at least 1 full year of employment and working at least halftime.	Burn-out: SMBQ. PA: adapted version of the 4-level Saltin Grimby Physical Activity Level Scale (reporting PA in the last 3 months). This scale makes a distinction between participants who are mostly sedentary, who engage in light PA for at least 2 h a week, who report at least 2 h per week of moderate PA or who engage in vigorous activity at least 5 h per week on several occasions.	More PA is associated with fewer symptoms of burn-out at a cross-sectional level at baseline ($r = -0.4$, $p < 0.01$). Individuals who became more active compared to others across the 6 years also showed a larger decrease in symptoms of burn-out ($r = -0.79$, $p < 0.01$).
Moueleu Ngalagou et al. [63] Cameroon	Cross-sectional	303 teaching staff members (lecturers, senior lecturers, professors): - 209 men, 94 women - Mean age: 43.0 ± 7.0 years	Burn-out: MBI. PA and sport practice: Ricci-Gagnon Questionnaire was used to assess the level of physical activities and sport practice.	Individuals reporting LPA or MVPA were significantly less likely to be classified as having elevated scores on burn-out compared to those who were inactive (LPA: OR, 0.13; 95% CI, 0.12–0.73); MVPA: OR, 0.14: 95% CI, 0.05–0.35).
Hu et al. [64] Taiwan	Cross-sectional	1560 full-time employees: - Mean age: 45.4 ± 8.9 years	Burn-out: CBI. It was not mentioned how physical inactivity was measured.	A positive correlation between physical inactivity and being in the upper tertile (range 37.5 to 100) of burn-out was found (lower tertile: 37.8% physically inactive, middle tertile: 38.4% physically inactive, upper tertile: 57.6% physically inactive; $p < 0.01$) (Upper vs. lower tertile: OR, 1.78; 95% CI, 1.33–2.37; $p < 0.01$).
Peterson et al. [65] Sweden	Cross-sectional	3719 employees (physicians, nurses, nursing assistants, social workers, occupational therapists, physiotherapists, psychologists, dental nurses, hygienists, dentists, administrators, teachers and technicians) in a Swedish Country Council: - 18% men, 82% women - Age range: between 22 and 66 years	Burn-out: OBI measuring 2 dimensions: exhaustion and disengagement. PA: frequency of physical exercise was assessed on a five-point scale scoring from 'never' to '3 times per week or more'. Exercising 2 times per week or more was classified as high, and 'never' and 'irregularly' was categorized as low PA.	Physical exercise played a minor role in discriminating between burn-out and non-burn-out groups: Emotional exhaustion and exercise: $r = 0.12$ (no p-value mentioned). Disengagement and exercise: $r = 0.04$ (no p-value mentioned).
Sane et al. [66] Iran	Cross-sectional	81 teachers of Danegaz University.	Burn-out: MBI. PA: Baecke's physical activity questionnaire	There is an inverse correlation between PA and burn-out ($r = -0.4$, $p = 0.001$).

Table 2. Cont.

Author (year) and Country	Design	Participants and Setting	Outcome Measure and Measurement Tools	Conclusion
Toker et al. [21] Israel	Longitudinal with 3 time points between 2003 and 2009.	1632 employees (working in high and low technology, teaching or academia, administration, sales and services, blue collar, health care): - 70% men, 30% women - Mean age: 46.6 ± 8.7 years - Working for minimum 50% (32% managerial position)	Burn-out: SMBQ. PA: based on patients' self-reports. Consistent with the American College of Sports Medicine and the American Heart Association guidelines, they were asked how many days per week and how many minutes each session they engaged over the past month in strenuous PA (activity that increases the heart rate and brings on a sweat) during their leisure time.	PA and burn-out are negatively correlated (job burn-out – PA T1: r = −0.10, p < 0.01; T2: r = −0.11, p < 0.01).
			Physical activity and sedentary behavior	
Jonsdottir et al. [67] Sweden	Longitudinal with 2 year follow-up (data was collected in 2004 and 2006)	3114 participants (health care workers and workers at the social insurance offices): - 420 men, 2694 women - Mean age: 49.0 ± 9.9 years - Only employees with at least 1 year employment and working at least 50% of a full-time equivalent.	Burn-out: SMBQ PA and sedentary behavior: adapted version of the 4-level Saltin Grimby Physical Activity Level Scale (reporting PA in the last 3 months). This scale makes a distinction between participants who are mostly sedentary, who engage in light PA for at least 2 h a week, who report at least 2 h per week of moderate PA or who engage in vigorous activity at least 5 h per week on several occasions.	Participation in LPA or MVPA was associated with lower reports of high burn-out levels (LPA: Prevalence Ratio, 0.61; 95% CI, 0.51–0.74; MVPA: Prevalence Ratio, 0.40; 95% CI 0.32–0.50). Individuals reporting LPA and MVPA at baseline were less likely to report burn-out at the follow-up compared to those reporting sedentary activity (LPA: PR, 0.59; 95% CI, 0.41–0.85; MVPA: PR, 0.43; 95% CI, 0.28–0.64).
Lindwall et al. [68] Sweden	Cross-sectional	177 employees (health care workers and workers at the social insurance offices): - 87 men, 90 women - Mean age: 39.1 ± 8.1 years - Only employees with at least 1 year employment and working at least 50% of a full-time equivalent.	Burn-out: SMBQ. PA: adapted version of the 4-level Saltin Grimby Physical Activity Level Scale (reporting PA in the last 3 months). This scale makes a distinction between participants who are mostly sedentary, who engage in light PA for at least 2 h a week, who report at least 2 h per week of moderate PA or who engage in vigorous activity at least 5 h per week on several occasions.	Individuals reporting LPA and MVPA were less likely to be classified as having elevated scores on burn-out compared to those who were sedentary (LPA: OR, 0.30; 95% CI, 0.12–0.73; MVPA: OR, 0.14; 95% CI, 0.05–0.35). No differences were found between the LPA and MVPA groups in terms of burn-out.

Table 2. *Cont.*

Author (year) and Country	Design	Participants and Setting	Outcome Measure and Measurement Tools	Conclusion
		Physical activity and dietary behavior		
Alexandrova-Karamanova [46] Greece, Portugal, Bulgaria, Romania, Turkey, Croatia and Macedonia	Cross-sectional	2623 health professionals working in university hospitals in Greece, Portugal, Bulgaria, Romania, Turkey, Croatia and Macedonia: - 24.5% men, 75.5% women - Mean age: 38.7 ± 10.2 years - 627 medical doctors, 1431 nurses, 565 residents	Burn-out: MBI-Human services survey PA and dietary behavior: Health Behaviors Questionnaire: PA and healthy eating were both assessed through a single item: "How many times do you exercise per week?" and "How many times in a week do you eat fast food?"	More frequent fast food consumption was significantly associated with higher emotional exhaustion and higher depersonalization (emotional exhaustion: $\beta = 0.14$; $p < 0.001$; depersonalization: $\beta = 0.16$; $p < 0.001$) and less frequent exercise (emotional exhaustion: $\beta = -0.17$; $p < 0.001$; depersonalization: $\beta = -0.12$; $p < 0.001$).
Gorter et al. [49] The Netherlands	Cross-sectional	709 dentists: - 594 men, 114 women - Mean age: 43.0 years (range: 21 – 62 years)	Burn-out: Dutch version of the MBI. PA and dietary behavior: Health behavior: Health behavior measured by 7 self-constructed items. An example of an item is: "To your opinion, do you eat healthy during work days?"	The high-risk group has a more unhealthy lifestyle, meaning that they perform less physical exercise and they consume less healthy diets during work days compared to the low-risk group (sporting/physical exercise: high-risk group: 28% several times a week; $p < 0.005$; Healthy diet at working days: high-risk group: 29% every day; $p < 0.005$).

Abbreviations: Maslach Burn-out Inventory (MBI), Shirom-Melamed Burn-out Questionnaire (SMBQ), The Oldenburg Burn-out Inventory (OBI), Copenhagen Burn-out Inventory (CBI), Physical Activity (PA) Low Physical Activity (LPA), Moderate-to-vigorous Physical activity (MVPA), Intervention Group (IG), Control Group (CG), Randomised Controlled Trial (RCT).

3.1. Physical Activity

All 25 studies assessed the relationship between physical activity and burn-out.

Nine out of ten experimental studies found a positive effect of physical activity on risk of burn-out. More specifically, five studies found a reduction in risk of burn-out in general (i.e., all three dimensions combined) due to physical activity (reduction ranging from 6.9% to 41.3%) [49,52–55]. Two studies assessed the effect of physical activity on all three dimensions of burn-out separately, reporting a positive effect on emotional exhaustion (−33.4% and −10%) and cynicism (−33.3% and −4%), but not on personal accomplishment [51,56]. However, one other study also assessed the effect of physical activity on emotional exhaustion, cynicism and personal accomplishment separately and did not find a significant effect on any dimension [50]. Two of the ten experimental studies assessed the effect of physical activity on emotional exhaustion only and showed a significant improvement in emotional exhaustion (−21.6% and −10%) [47,48].

Four experimental studies also conducted follow-up measurements, with three studies reporting a decrease in risk of burn-out three and six months after the physical activity intervention [47,53,56]. The fourth study equally showed a decrease after six months and this maintained after 12 months [52]. Four studies compared physical activity interventions with other interventions such as multimodal rehabilitation and basic care, but no significant differences in the decrease in burn-out risk between these interventions were reported [49,52,54,56].

All 15 observational studies assessed the relationship between physical activity and risk of burn-out, or one of its components. Fourteen observational studies found a negative association between physical activity and risk of burn-out, or one of its components, and one did not find a relationship. More specifically, ten studies assessed the relationship between physical activity and risk of burn-out generally [21,61,63,64,66–69], of which nine found a negative association and one did not find a significant relation between both [65]. One observational study assessed both the relationship between physical activity and risk of burn-out and all three dimensions separately and found negative associations between physical activity and risk of burn-out, emotional exhaustion and cynicism and a positive association between physical activity and professional efficacy [57]. Four other studies found a negative association between physical activity and emotional exhaustion [46,58,60,70] and one of them also found a positive association between physical activity and cynicism [46]. Lastly, one of 15 observational studies concluded that the association between physical activity and risk of burn-out was stronger in workers with a sedentary job [58].

3.2. Sedentary Behavior

Two of the 15 observational studies including physical activity also assessed the relationship between sedentary behavior and risk of burn-out. Both studies found a positive association with risk of burn-out [67,68].

3.3. Dietary Behavior

Besides physical activity, two of the observational studies also examined the link between diet and risk of burn-out. In both studies diet was measured by a single question. The study by Alexandrova-Karamanova et al. [46] measured fast food consumption by asking how many times in a week people ate fast food, and concluded that fast food consumption was positively associated with risk of burn-out. In the study by Gorter et al. [69] dietary behavior was measured by asking how many healthy diets participants consumed during workdays, and found that the amount of healthy diets during workdays and the risk of burn-out were negatively associated.

3.4. Quality Assessment of the Included Studies

According to the "Standard quality assessment criteria for evaluating primary research papers from a variety of fields" [45], the mean article quality score was 0.82 ± 0.10 out of a total of 1 (Table 3). Eleven articles scored below the mean score with a minimum score of 0.61. Fourteen articles scored above the mean score with a maximum score of 0.95.

Table 3. Quality assessment of the included studies.

	Research Question	Study Design	Method	Subject	Allocation	Blinding of Investigators	Blinding of Subjects	Outcome	Sample Size	Analytic Methods	Estimate of Variance	Confounding	Results	Conclusions	Summary Score (/1)
Experiment studies															
Physical activity															
de Vries et al. [47]	2	2	1	2	2	0	0	2	2	2	2	2	2	2	0.82
Dreyer et al. [48]	2	1	1	2	1	0	0	1	1	2	2	0	2	2	0.61
Eskilsson et al. [49]	2	2	1	2	1	0	N/A	2	1	2	2	0	2	2	0.81
Freitas et al. [50]	2	1	1	2	N/A	0	N/A	1	0	2	2	0	2	2	0.63
Gerber et al. [51]	1	1	1	2	N/A	0	N/A	2	2	2	2	2	2	2	0.79
Heiden et al. [52]	1	2	1	2	1	0	0	1	1	2	2	2	2	2	0.68
Lindegard et al. [53]	2	1	1	2	N/A	0	N/A	2	1	2	2	2	2	2	0.79
Stenlund et al. [54]	2	2	1	2	2	0	0	2	1	2	2	2	2	2	0.79
Tsai et al. [55]	2	2	1	2	0	0	0	2	2	2	2	2	2	2	0.75
Van Rhenen et al. [56]	1	2	1	2	1	0	0	2	1	2	2	2	2	2	0.71
Observational studies															
Physical activity															
Ahola et al. [57]	2	1	1	2	N/A	N/A	N/A	2	2	2	2	N/A	2	2	0.90
Bernaards et al. [58]	2	2	1	1	N/A	N/A	N/A	2	1	2	2	2	2	2	0.86
Carson et al. [59]	2	1	1	2	N/A	N/A	N/A	2	2	1	2	N/A	2	2	0.85
de Vries et al. [60]	2	2	1	2	N/A	N/A	N/A	2	2	2	2	2	2	2	0.95
Hu et al. [64]	2	2	1	2	N/A	N/A	N/A	1	1	2	2	N/A	2	2	0.85
Liang et al. [61]	2	1	1	2	N/A	N/A	N/A	2	1	2	2	1	2	2	0.82
Lindwall et al. [62]	1	2	1	2	N/A	N/A	N/A	2	1	2	2	2	2	2	0.86
Moueleu Ngalagou et al. [63]	2	2	1	2	N/A	N/A	N/A	2	2	2	2	N/A	2	2	0.95
Peterson et al. [65]	2	2	1	1	N/A	N/A	N/A	2	2	2	2	N/A	2	2	0.9
Sane et al. [66]	1	1	1	0	N/A	N/A	N/A	1	1	2	2	N/A	2	2	0.65
Toker et al. [21]	2	2	1	2	N/A	N/A	N/A	2	1	2	2	2	2	2	0.91

Table 3. *Cont.*

	Research Question	Study Design	Method	Subject	Allocation	Blinding of Investigators	Blinding of Subjects	Outcome	Sample Size	Analytic Methods	Estimate of Variance	Confounding	Results	Conclusions	Summary Score (/1)
Physical activity and sedentary behavior															
Jonsdottir et al. [67]	2	2	1	2	N/A	N/A	N/A	2	2	2	2	2	2	2	0.95
Lindwall et al. [68]	2	2	1	2	N/A	N/A	N/A	2	1	2	2	2	2	2	0.91
Physical activity and dietary behavior															
Alexandrova-Karamanova et al. [46]	2	2	1	2	N/A	N/A	N/A	1	2	2	2	2	2	2	0.91
Gorter et al. [69]	1	1	1	1	N/A	N/A	N/A	2	2	2	2	N/A	2	2	0.80

4. Discussion

In this systematic review, an overview of studies investigating the association between energy balance-related behavior and burn-out is provided. In total, 25 studies were found, of which 21 assessed the relationship between physical activity and risk of burn-out, two studies investigated the association between physical activity, sedentary behavior and the risk of burn-out, and two assessed the link between physical activity, dietary behavior and risk of burn-out. No articles using a holistic approach—i.e., investigating the relationship between energy balance and energy balance-related behavior as a whole and risk of burn-out—were found. Nevertheless, it is important to use a combined approach to gain more insight regarding, e.g., which behavior may have a bigger impact on burn-out risk. Moreover, as previously mentioned, van der Ploeg et al. [27] indicated that sedentary behavior and physical (in)activity should be targeted at the same time in public health strategies. The present systematic review, for example, shows that the association between physical activity and risk of burn-out was stronger in workers with a sedentary job, showing a possible interaction between both physical activity and sedentary behavior in relation to burn-out risk [58]. A similar interaction between both behaviors, but with mortality as the outcome measure, was found in a large-scale meta-analysis (including over one million men and women), where high levels of moderate intensity physical activity (about 60–75 min per day) eliminated the increased risk of death associated with high sitting time [71]. In addition, previous studies showed that increased screen time was associated with an overall poor diet quality [72,73]. The above indicates possible triangular interactions, again highlighting the importance of combining all energy balance-related behaviors when investigating their association with burn-out risk.

Furthermore, despite the fact that no studies investigating the relationship between energy balance (i.e., energy intake vs. energy expenditure [74]) and burn-out were found, a positive or negative energy balance may also be associated with burn-out. The interaction and co-existence of energy balance-related behaviors determine whether or not a positive or negative energy balance is experienced [75]. As energy imbalances may lead to the development of overweight and obesity (= physical health) [74], one may hypothesize that a similar imbalance may lead to decreased mental health as well. Previous research, in fact, demonstrates that obesity is associated with higher levels of burn-out [76].

Despite the heterogeneity of populations, assessment methods for both risk of burn-out and physical activity, and physical activity interventions, the vast majority of the experimental studies, including 5 RCTs, concluded that physical activity is effective in reducing the risk of burn-out, suggesting a causal link between both. The experimental studies showed a decrease in burn-out risk ranging from 6.9% to 41.3% [49,52–55], a decrease in emotional exhaustion between 10% and 33.4% [47,48,51,56] and a decrease in cynicism of 33.3% and 4% [48,51]. One experimental study by Freitas et al. [50], showing a relatively low quality score of 0.63, did not find any significant effect of physical activity on risk of burn-out. This may be due to the small sample size ($n = 21$) and the duration of the physical activities performed in this study. The participants had to perform a 10-min workplace physical activity session on weekdays (no information on type or intensity was provided), while the World Health Organization (WHO) [16] recommends that adults should be physically active at a moderate intensity for at least 150 min per week or at a vigorous intensity for at least 75 min per week or an equivalent combination of both moderate and vigorous intensity activity. So, the total duration of the physical activities performed in the study by Freitas et al. [50] (ten minutes per day, for five days a week) was not meeting the above guidelines [77]. On the other hand, the study by Stenlund et al. [54], in which the performed physical activities (60 min, twice a week, at a moderate intensity) also failed to meet the WHO guidelines, did report a significant effect of physical activity on burn-out. It should be mentioned that, despite not meeting the recommendations, total physical activity duration in the latter study was still much higher compared to the study by Freitas et al. [50] (i.e., 120 min versus 50 min per week, respectively). In another experimental study [55], two groups of participants performed high- and low-intensive physical activities, respectively, for 60 min twice a week (=120 min in total). The low intensive group also failed to meet the WHO guidelines. Nevertheless, both groups (high vs. low intensity) had more or less the same effect on burn-out (reductions of 8.1% and 8.2%, respectively) [55]. These findings suggest that lower (than recommended) amounts of physical activity of 120 min per week (at a low to moderate intensity) may already be effective in reducing burn-out risk. Furthermore, the role of intensity may be questioned. It should be mentioned, however, that the physical activities performed in the other experimental studies (showing a positive effect of physical activity on burn-out risk) were in line with the WHO guidelines, as they lasted 20 to 60 min for two to five times per week at a moderate to vigorous intensity [47–49,51,53]. The remaining two experimental studies did not give clear information about the duration of the physical activity sessions [52,56]. Further, four experimental studies [47,52,53,56] also conducted follow-up measurements and showed a decrease in risk of burn-out three, six and 12 months after the interventions, indicating long-term effectiveness, even when the physical activity intervention did not remain in place.

Our results are in line with the systematic review by Naczenski et al. [1] showing strong evidence for the effect of physical activity on reducing (emotional) exhaustion, but limited evidence for the effect on professional efficacy and cynicism. Further, Naczenski et al. [1] concluded that being physically active one or two times per week for four to 18 weeks has promising effects on reducing burn-out symptoms. The present systematic review slightly deviates from this conclusion, showing that positive effects on burn-out risk were achieved when being physically active two to five times per week for 20 to 60 min, for six to 18 weeks, with 18 weeks showing the biggest reduction in burn-out risk (−47.8%) [53]. The latter suggests that the longer the duration of the physical activity intervention, the higher the reduction in burn-out risk. However, due to the large variety in type, intensity, duration and frequency of the performed physical activities in the included studies, comparison of the effectiveness of the individual interventions remains difficult. Further research to unravel the respective effects of type, intensity, duration and frequency is therefore highly recommended. Furthermore, to better understand the relationship between physical activity and burn-out risk, it is also important to investigate the underlying physiological mechanisms. For example, the role of BDNF might be interesting as BDNF-levels increase when physical activity is performed, while on the other hand, BDNF-levels were found to be decreased in people having burn-out [22]. Four experimental studies [49,52,54,56] compared physical activity interventions with other interventions—such as basic care, cognitive interventions and a multimodal rehabilitation program—and did not find physical activity to be more effective compared to the other treatment arms. It should be mentioned that, in one of these studies [52], the aforementioned conclusion was based on the results of six and 12 months after the intervention was completed, possibly causing differences between treatment effects to have been diminished. Another possible reason for these results may be a shared effect between the interventions, resulting in no effect of intervention type [78]. As suggested by Heiden et al. [52], the same (psychosocial) attention was given to all patients in both interventions, suggesting (psychosocial) attention to be such a shared effect. Furthermore, as human interaction was also present in the other experimental studies (e.g., interaction between the researcher or therapist and the participant during the intervention phase), part of the intervention effects might be explained by the same psychosocial component [49,52,54,56].

These results might suggest that physical activity may be equally effective compared to other types of interventions, as long as there is a psychosocial component involved. Future research should further unravel the relative importance of physical activity versus other intervention components when aiming at reducing burn-out risk.

Regarding sedentary behavior, only positive relationships with risk of burn-out were reported, indicating that higher levels of sedentary behavior are associated with higher burn-out risk. It should be mentioned, however, that only two observational studies [62,67] were found, making it difficult to draw any firm conclusions. Nevertheless, the quality score of these two studies was high (0.86 and 0.95). Besides, it is important to mention that these studies primarily aimed to assess the relationship between physical activity and risk of burn-out. In both studies, the assessment method of physical activity was the 4-level Saltin Grimby Physical Activity Level Scale [79], of which the lowest level reflects sedentary behavior. This level means that participants were not participating in any leisure-time physical activities or sport activities, which is not in line with the definition of sedentary behavior [25]. Furthermore, no validated objective (e.g., inclinometers, accelerometers) nor subjective (e.g., more detailed context-specific questionnaires) assessment methods for sedentary behavior were used. Despite the fact that sedentary behavior may influence mental health and despite its impact on the risk of the occurrence of common mental disorders such as depression, decreased mood and anxiety, no experimental studies investigating the influence of sedentary behavior on burn-out risk were found. Furthermore, the study by Bernaards et al. [58] concluded that the association between physical activity and burn-out risk was stronger in workers with a sedentary job. This suggests a possible moderating role of sedentary behavior in the physical activity-burn-out risk relationship pathway. So, the interaction between physical activity and sedentary behavior should be further investigated while explaining burn-out risk.

Two observational studies [46,69], with quality scores of 0.80 and 0.91 respectively, found that a healthier diet is related to a lower risk of burn-out. Because only two studies were found and the fact that these two studies were investigating different aspects of dietary behavior, namely fast food consumption and the amount of healthy diets during work days, it is difficult to draw reliable conclusions regarding this relationship. Moreover, these two studies did not use valid and reliable assessment methods to measure both aspects. Alexandrova-Karamanova et al. [46] measured fast food consumption by one single self-constructed question, namely "How many times in a week do you eat fast food?". In the study by Gorter et al. [69] dietary behavior was measured by asking how many healthy diets participants consumed during workdays, while "healthy diets" was not defined. These methodological shortcomings make it even more difficult to draw firm conclusions.

It has been shown that diet may influence mental health. A systematic review and meta-analysis by Tolkien et al. [80] for example, concluded that an anti-inflammatory diet may play an important role in preventing or reducing depression risk and symptoms. Moreover, because of the link between burn-out and neurotransmission and the role diet may play herein, it is important to further investigate the link between dietary behavior and burn-out risk by conducting experimental research using valid and reliable assessment methods (e.g., food diaries, 24-hour recalls or food frequency questionnaires).

Because all studies regarding sedentary behavior, dietary behavior and burn-out risk had an observational design, no conclusions about the causal relationship can be made. As hypothesized above, being sedentary may increase the risk of burn-out through different physiological mechanisms, while a burn-out may also cause people to be more sedentary, and so reversed causality is possible. The same may be true for dietary behavior. This shows the need for more experimental studies investigating the causal relationship between sedentary and dietary behavior and burn-out risk.

There are several limitations to the included studies. A first limitation is the fact that some studies [57,58,69] measured physical activity with only one or two single self-constructed questions. Moreover, some measurement methods for physical activity had methodological shortcomings. The study by Liang et al. [61], for example, measured exercise behavior on a 5-point scale with anchors 1: 'never' to 5: 'many times in a week', while 'many times' was not defined. Future research should use validated questionnaires (e.g., International Physical Activity Questionnaire [81]), and preferably objective measures, such as accelerometers or pedometers. The same can be said for sedentary and dietary behavior. A second limitation is that less than half of the included studies used the Maslach Burnout Inventory (MBI), while the MBI is the gold standard assessment tool for burn-out [82]. All the other assessment tools for burn-out used in the included studies are based on other definitions of burn-out and are mostly measuring one dimension, namely (emotional) exhaustion. It is recommended that future research uses the gold standard assessment tool for measuring burn-out, in order to increase measurement homogeneity across studies. A third limitation is that some studies are mixing up the terms "physical inactivity" and "sedentary behavior". Two of the included studies [57,63] use a physical activity questionnaire to classify people as active or inactive, and considered inactive people to be sedentary, while literature clearly shows that physical inactivity and sedentary behavior are two different concepts [27,28,83]. A fourth limitation is that the majority of the included studies did not take physiological, psychological and sociological confounders into account, and so conclusions may have to be interpreted with caution. A fifth limitation is that most studies consisted mostly of female participants, which may have influenced the results. Research shows that women generally eat healthier but are less physically active compared to men [84–89]. Moreover, a meta-analysis showed that women are more likely to report burn-out [90]. More specifically, women reported to be more emotionally exhausted than men, while men were more depersonalized [90]. Hence, future studies investigating the association between energy balance-related behavior and burn-out should take sex into account. Lastly, some articles were missing some relevant information, such as how physical inactivity was measured, so the authors had to be contacted. Unfortunately, we did not always get a response leaving some queries unanswered.

There are also a few limitations to the present systematic review. Since non-English written publications were excluded, we may have missed out on important scientific articles in other languages. Additionally, the used quality assessment tool does not distinguish between experimental and observational studies. Experimental studies can be considered higher in quality and so they should receive a higher score in the quality assessment. However, when calculating the mean quality score per study design, a higher mean quality score of 0.87 ± 0.08 for the observational studies was found, compared to a mean quality score of 0.74 ± 0.08 among the experimental studies.

A strength of this systematic review is the fact that this is the first systematic review aiming to include articles of all study designs investigating the relationship between energy balance-related behavior as a whole (i.e., the combination of physical activity, sedentary behavior and dietary behavior) and burn-out risk. As—in the present review—no studies using this holistic approach were found, and because of the hypothesized role these three components may play in reducing or preventing burn-out, further research on this topic is needed.

5. Conclusions

This systematic review shows that any type of physical activity, lasting 20 to 60 min and performed two to five times per week for six to 18 weeks, may be effective in reducing the risk of burn-out. The few observational studies linking sedentary and dietary behavior with burn-out risk suggest that engaging in frequent sedentary behavior and eating less healthy are each associated with higher burn-out risk. More high-quality research is needed to unravel the causal relationship between sedentary and dietary behavior and the risk of burn-out.

Author Contributions: This work was carried out in collaboration between the authors Y.V., K.D.M., E.V.D.L., E.V.H., E.Z. and T.D. Y.V., K.D.M., E.V.H., E.Z. and T.D. designed the study. Y.V. performed the literature search, data extraction, data-analysis and drafted the manuscript. E.V.D.L. conducted the literature search and participated in the data extraction and data-analysis. K.D.M., E.V.H., E.Z. and T.D. provided guidance about the content of the review and contributed to multiple revisions of the manuscript. All authors read and approved the final manuscript.

Funding: This research received no external funding.

Acknowledgments: We thank Katrien Alewaeters, the head of the university library, for reviewing the methodology of the search and selection process of this systematic review.

Conflicts of Interest: The authors declare that they have no conflict of interests.

References

1. Naczenski, L.M.; De Vries, J.D.; Van Hooff, M.L.M.; Kompier, M.A.J. Systematic review of the association between physical activity and burnout. *J. Occup. Heal.* **2017**, *59*, 477–494. [CrossRef] [PubMed]
2. Leka, S.; Jain, A.; World Health Organization. *Health Impact of Psychosocial Hazards at Work: An Overview*; World Health Organization: Geneva, Switzerland, 2010.
3. Ferreira, A.I.; Martinez, L.F. Presenteeism and burnout among teachers in public and private Portuguese elementary schools. *Int. J. Hum. Resour. Manag.* **2012**, *23*, 4380–4390. [CrossRef]

4. Harvey, E.; Burns, J. Staff burnout and absenteeism through service transition: From hospital to hostel. *Ment. Handicap Res.* **1994**, *7*, 328–337. [CrossRef]

5. Wallace, J.E.; Lemaire, J.B.; Ghali, W.A. Physician wellness: A missing quality indicator. *Lancet* **2009**, *374*, 1714–1721. [CrossRef]

6. Ochentel, O.; Humphrey, C.; Pfeifer, K. Efficacy of Exercise Therapy in Persons with Burnout. A Systematic Review and Meta-Analysis. *J. Sports Sci. Med.* **2018**, *17*, 475–484.

7. Rowe, D.S. The Stress Burden: Strategies for Management. Available online: https://www.thefreelibrary.com/The+stress+burden%3a+strategies+for+management.-a0288874874 (accessed on 4 October 2019).

8. EU-OSHA. *Calculating the Cost of Work-Related Stress and Psychosocial Risks*; Publications Office of the European Union: Luxembourg, 2014.

9. Maslach, C.; Schaufeli, W.B.; Leiter, M.P. Job Burnout. *Annu. Rev. Psychol.* **2001**, *52*, 397–422. [CrossRef]

10. Schaufeli, W.B.; Leiter, M.P.; Maslach, C. Burnout: 35 years of research and practice. *Career Dev. Int.* **2009**, *14*, 204–220. [CrossRef]

11. Guan, S.; Xiaerfuding, X.; Ning, L.; Lian, Y.; Jiang, Y.; Liu, J.; Ng, T.B. Effect of Job Strain on Job Burnout, Mental Fatigue and Chronic Diseases among Civil Servants in the Xinjiang Uygur Autonomous Region of China. *Int. J. Environ. Res. Public Heal.* **2017**, *14*, 872. [CrossRef]

12. Awa, W.L.; Plaumann, M.; Walter, U. Burnout prevention: A review of intervention programs. *Patient Educ. Couns.* **2010**, *78*, 184–190. [CrossRef]

13. Melnyk, B.M.; Jacobson, D.; Kelly, S.; O'Haver, J.; Small, L.; Mays, M.Z. Improving the Mental Health, Healthy Lifestyle Choices, and Physical Health of Hispanic Adolescents: A Randomized Controlled Pilot Study. *J. Sch. Heal.* **2009**, *79*, 575–584. [CrossRef]

14. Jacka, F.N.; Mykletun, A.; Berk, M. Moving towards a population health approach to the primary prevention of common mental disorders. *BMC Med.* **2012**, *10*, 149. [CrossRef]

15. Lucas, M.; Mekary, R.; Pan, A.; Mirzaei, F.; O'Reilly, É.J.; Willett, W.C.; Koenen, K.; Okereke, O.I.; Ascherio, A. Relation Between Clinical Depression Risk and Physical Activity and Time Spent Watching Television in Older Women: A 10-Year Prospective Follow-up Study. *Am. J. Epidemiol.* **2011**, *174*, 1017–1027. [CrossRef] [PubMed]

16. WHO. *Global Recommendations on Physical Activity for Health*; World Health Organization: Geneva, Switzerland, 2010; Volume 60, pp. 1–58.

17. Ainslie, P.N.; Cotter, J.D.; George, K.P.; Lucas, S.; Murrell, C.; Shave, R.; Thomas, K.N.; Williams, M.J.A.; Atkinson, G. Elevation in cerebral blood flow velocity with aerobic fitness throughout healthy human ageing. *J. Physiol.* **2008**, *586*, 4005–4010. [CrossRef]

18. Colcombe, S.J.; Kramer, A.F.; Erickson, K.I.; Scalf, P.; McAuley, E.; Cohen, N.J.; Webb, A.; Jerome, G.J.; Marquez, D.X.; Elavsky, S. Cardiovascular fitness, cortical plasticity, and aging. *Proc. Natl. Acad. Sci. USA* **2004**, *101*, 3316–3321. [CrossRef]

19. Erickson, K.I.; Voss, M.W.; Prakash, R.S.; Basak, C.; Szabo, A.; Chaddock, L.; Kim, J.S.; Heo, S.; Alves, H.; White, S.M.; et al. Exercise training increases size of hippocampus and improves memory. *Proc. Natl. Acad. Sci. USA* **2011**, *108*, 3017–3022. [CrossRef]

20. Sonnentag, S. *Psychological Detachment from Work During Leisure Time: The Benefits of Mentally Disengaging from Work*; Psychological Science: Mannheim, Germany, 2012; Volume 21, pp. 114, 118.

21. Toker, S.; Biron, M. Job burnout and depression: Unraveling their temporal relationship and considering the role of physical activity. *J. Appl. Psychol.* **2012**, *97*, 699–710. [CrossRef]

22. He, S.; Zhang, Y.; Zhan, J.; Wang, C.; Du, X.; Yin, G.; Cao, B.; Ning, Y.; Soares, J.; Zhang, X. Burnout and cognitive impairment: Associated with serum BDNF in a Chinese Han population. *Psychoneuroendocrinology* **2017**, *77*, 236–243. [CrossRef]

23. Schwarzer, R.; Hallum, S. Perceived Teacher Self-Efficacy as a Predictor of Job Stress and Burnout: Mediation Analyses. *Appl. Psychol.* **2008**, *57*, 152–171. [CrossRef]

24. Westman, M.; Etzion, D. The impact of vacation and job stress on burnout and absenteeism. *Psychol. Heal.* **2001**, *16*, 595–606. [CrossRef]

25. Barnes, J.; Behrens, T.K.; Benden, M.E.; Biddle, S.; Bond, D.; Brassard, P. Letter to the editor: Standardized use of the terms "sedentary" and "sedentary behaviours". *Appl. Physiol. Nutr. Metab.* **2012**, *37*, 540–542. [CrossRef]

26. Mansoubi, M.; Pearson, N.; Biddle, S.J.; Clemes, S. The relationship between sedentary behaviour and physical activity in adults: A systematic review. *Prev. Med.* **2014**, *69*, 28–35. [CrossRef] [PubMed]

27. van der Ploeg, H.P.; Hillsdon, M. Is sedentary behaviour just physical inactivity by another name? *Int. J. Behav. Nutr. Phys. Act.* **2017**, *14*, 142. [CrossRef] [PubMed]

28. Panahi, S.; Tremblay, A. Sedentariness and Health: Is Sedentary Behavior More Than Just Physical Inactivity? *Front. Public Health* **2018**, *6*, 258. [CrossRef] [PubMed]

29. De Rezende, L.F.M.; Lopes, M.R.; Rey-Lopez, J.P.; Matsudo, V.K.R.; Luiz, O.D.C. Sedentary Behavior and Health Outcomes: An Overview of Systematic Reviews. *PLoS ONE* **2014**, *9*, e105620. [CrossRef] [PubMed]

30. Hoang, T.D.; Reis, J.; Zhu, N.; Jacobs, D.R.; Launer, L.J.; Whitmer, R.A.; Sidney, S.; Yaffe, K. Effect of Early Adult Patterns of Physical Activity and Television Viewing on Midlife Cognitive Function. *JAMA Psychiatry* **2016**, *73*, 73–79. [CrossRef] [PubMed]

31. Kesse-Guyot, E.; Charreire, H.; Andreeva, V.A.; Touvier, M.; Hercberg, S.; Galan, P.; Oppert, J.M. Cross-sectional and longitudinal associations of different sedentary behaviors with cognitive performance in older adults. *PLoS ONE* **2012**, *7*. [CrossRef]

32. Engeroff, T.; Fuzeki, E.; Vogt, L.; Fleckenstein, J.; Schwarz, S.; Matura, S.; Pilatus, U.; Deichmann, R.; Hellweg, R.; Pantel, J.; et al. Is Objectively Assessed Sedentary Behavior, Physical Activity and Cardiorespiratory Fitness Linked to Brain Plasticity Outcomes in Old Age? *Neuroscience* **2018**, *388*, 384–392. [CrossRef]

33. Teychenne, M.; Ball, K.; Salmon, J. Sedentary Behavior and Depression Among Adults: A Review. *Int. J. Behav. Med.* **2010**, *17*, 246–254. [CrossRef]

34. Endrighi, R.; Steptoe, A.; Hamer, M. The effect of experimentally induced sedentariness on mood and psychobiological responses to mental stress. *Br. J. Psychiatry* **2016**, *208*, 245–251. [CrossRef]

35. Tops, M.; Boksem, M.A.; Wijers, A.A.; van Duinen, H.; Den Boer, J.A.; Meijman, T.F.; Korf, J. The psychobiology of burnout: Are there two different syndromes? *Neuropsychobiology* **2007**, *55*, 143–150. [CrossRef]

36. Yao, Y.; Zhao, S.; Zhang, Y.; Tang, L.; An, Z.; Lu, L.; Yao, S. Job-related burnout is associated with brain neurotransmitter levels in Chinese medical workers: A cross-sectional study. *J. Int. Med. Res.* **2018**, *46*, 3226–3235. [CrossRef] [PubMed]

37. Marriott, B.M. (Ed.) *Food Components to Enhance Performance: An Evaluation of Potential Performance-Enhancing Food Components for Operational Rations*; National Academic Press: Washington, DC, USA, 1994.

38. Dye, L.; Lluch, A.; Blundell, J.E. Macronutrients and mental performance. *Nutrition* **2000**, *16*, 1021–1034. [CrossRef]

39. Kaplan, R.J.; Greenwood, C.E.; Winocur, G.; Wolever, T.M. Cognitive performance is associated with glucose regulation in healthy elderly persons and can be enhanced with glucose and dietary carbohydrates. *Am. J. Clin. Nutr.* **2000**, *72*, 825–836. [CrossRef] [PubMed]

40. Kennedy, D.O.; Scholey, A. Glucose administration, heart rate and cognitive performance: Effects of increasing mental effort. *Psychopharmacology* **2000**, *149*, 63–71. [CrossRef] [PubMed]

41. Chung, Y.C.; Park, C.H.; Kwon, H.K.; Park, Y.M.; Kim, Y.S.; Doo, J.K.; Shin, D.H.; Jung, E.S.; Oh, M.R.; Chae, S.W. Improved cognitive performance following supplementation with a mixed-grain diet in high school students: A randomized controlled trial. *Nutrition* **2012**, *28*, 165–172. [CrossRef] [PubMed]

42. Fontani, G.; Corradeschi, F.; Felici, A.; Alfatti, F.; Bugarini, R.; Fiaschi, A.I.; Cerretani, D.; Montorfano, G.; Rizzo, A.M.; Berra, B. Blood profiles, body fat and mood state in healthy subjects on different diets supplemented with Omega-3 polyunsaturated fatty acids. *Eur. J. Clin. Investig.* **2005**, *35*, 499–507. [CrossRef] [PubMed]

43. Moher, D.; Liberati, A.; Tetzlaff, J.; Altman, D.G.; PRISMA Group. Preferred Reporting Items for Systematic Reviews and Meta-Analyses: The PRISMA Statement. *Ann. Intern. Med.* **2009**, *151*, 264–269. [CrossRef]

44. da Costa Santos, C.M.; de Mattos Pimenta, C.A.; Nobre, M.R. The PICO strategy for the research question construction and evidence search. *Rev. Latino-Americana de Enferm.* **2017**, *15*, 508–511. [CrossRef]

45. Kmet, L.M.; Cook, L.S.; Lee, R.C. Standard Quality Assessment Criteria for Evaluating Primary Research Papers from a Variety of Fields. *HTA Initiative* **2004**, *2*, 1–31.

46. Alexandrova-Karamanova, A.; Todorova, I.; Montgomery, A.; Panagopoulou, E.; Costa, P.; Băban, A.; Davas, A.; Milošević, M.; Mijakoski, D. Burnout and health behaviors in health professionals from seven European countries. *Int. Arch. Occup. Environ. Heal.* **2016**, *89*, 1059–1075. [CrossRef]

47. De Vries, J.D.; Van Hooff, M.L.; Guerts, S.A.; Kompier, M.A.; Jd, D.V.; Mlm, V.H.; Sae, G.; Maj, K. Exercise to reduce work-related fatigue among employees: A randomized controlled trial. *Scand. J. Work. Environ. Heal.* **2017**, *43*, 337–349. [CrossRef]

48. Dreyer, S.; Dreyer, L.; Rankin, D. Effects of a 10-week High-Intensity Exercise Intervention on College Staff with Psychological Burnout and Multiple Risk Facts. *J. Res.* **2012**, *7*, 27–33.

49. Eskilsson, T.; Järvholm, L.S.; Gavelin, H.M.; Neely, A.S.; Boraxbekk, C.-J. Aerobic training for improved memory in patients with stress-related exhaustion: A randomized controlled trial. *BMC Psychiatry* **2017**, *17*, 322. [CrossRef]

50. Freitas, A.R.; Carneseca, E.C.; Paiva, C.E.; Paiva, B.S.R. Impact of a physical activity program on the anxiety, depression, occupational stress and burnout syndrome of nursing professionals1. *Rev. Latino-Americana de Enferm.* **2014**, *22*, 332–336. [CrossRef]

51. Gerber, M.; Brand, S.; Elliot, C.; Holsboer-Trachsler, E.; Pühse, U.; Beck, J. Aerobic exercise training and burnout: A pilot study with male participants suffering from burnout. *BMC Res. Notes* **2013**, *6*, 78. [CrossRef]

52. Heiden, M.; Lyskov, E.; Nakata, M.; Sahlin, K.; Sahlin, T.; Barnekow-Bergkvist, M. Evaluation of cognitive behavioural training and physical activity for patients with stress-related illnesses: A randomized controlled study. *Acta Derm. Venereol.* **2007**, *39*, 366–373. [CrossRef]

53. Lindegård, A.; Jonsdottir, I.H.; Börjesson, M.; Lindwall, M.; Gerber, M. Changes in mental health in compliers and non-compliers with physical activity recommendations in patients with stress-related exhaustion. *BMC Psychiatry* **2015**, *15*, 272. [CrossRef]

54. Stenlund, T.; Birgander, L.S.; Lindahl, B.; Nilsson, L.; Ahlgren, C. Effects of Qigong in patients with burnout: A randomized controlled trial. *J. Rehabil. Med.* **2009**, *41*, 761–767. [CrossRef]

55. Tsai, H.H.; Yeh, C.Y.; Su, C.T.; Chen, C.J.; Peng, S.M.; Chen, R.Y. The effects of exercise program on burnout and metabolic syndrome components in banking and insurance workers. *Ind. Heal.* **2013**, *51*, 336–346. [CrossRef]

56. Van Rhenen, W.; Blonk, R.W.B.; Van Der Klink, J.J.L.; Van Dijk, F.J.H.; Schaufeli, W.B. The effect of a cognitive and a physical stress-reducing programme on psychological complaints. *Int. Arch. Occup. Environ. Heal.* **2005**, *78*, 139–148. [CrossRef]

57. Ahola, K.; Pulkki-Raback, L.; Kouvonen, A.; Rossi, H.; Aromaa, A.; Lonnqvist, J. Burnout and behavior-related health risk factors: Results from the population-based Finnish Health 2000 study. *J. Occup. Environ. Med.* **2012**, *54*, 17–22. [CrossRef]

58. Bernaards, C.M.; Jans, M.P.; van den Heuvel, S.G.; Hendriksen, I.J.; Houtman, I.L.; Bongers, P.M. Can strenuous leisure time physical activity prevent psychological complaints in a working population? *Occup. Environ. Med.* **2006**, *63*, 10–16. [CrossRef]

59. Carson, R.L.; Baumgartner, J.J.; Matthews, R.A.; Tsouloupas, C.N. Emotional exhaustion, absenteeism, and turnover intentions in childcare teachers: Examining the impact of physical activity behaviors. *J. Health Psychol.* **2010**, *15*, 905–914. [CrossRef]

60. de Vries, J.D.; Claessens, B.J.C.; van Hooff, M.L.M.; Geurts, S.A.E.; van den Bossche, S.N.J.; Kompier, M.A.J. Disentangling longitudinal relations between physical activity, work-related fatigue, and task demands. *Int. Arch. Occup. Environ. Health* **2016**, *89*, 89–101. [CrossRef]

61. Liang, H.-L.; Kao, Y.-T.; Lin, C.-C. Moderating effect of regulatory focus on burnout and exercise behavior. *Percept. Mot. Skills* **2013**, *117*, 696–708. [CrossRef]

62. Lindwall, M.; Gerber, M.; Jonsdottir, I.H.; Börjesson, M.; Ahlborg, G., Jr. The relationships of change in physical activity with change in depression, anxiety, and burnout: A longitudinal study of Swedish healthcare workers. *Health Psychol.* **2014**, *33*, 1309–1318. [CrossRef]

63. Moueleu Ngalagou, P.T.; Assomo-Ndemba, P.B.; Owona Manga, L.J.; Owoundi Ebolo, H.; Ayina Ayina, C.N.; Lobe Tanga, M.Y.; Guessogo, W.R.; Mekoulou Ndongo, J.; Temfemo, A.; Mandengue, S.H. Burnout syndrome and associated factors among university teaching staff in Cameroon: Effect of the practice of sport and physical activities and leisures. *Encephale* **2018**. [CrossRef]

64. Hu, N.-C.; Chen, J.-D.; Cheng, T.-J. The associations between long working hours, physical inactivity, and burnout. *J. Occup. Environ. Med.* **2016**, *58*, 514–518. [CrossRef]

65. Peterson, U.; Demerouti, E.; Bergstrom, G.; Samuelsson, M.; Asberg, M.; Nygren, A. Burnout and physical and mental health among Swedish healthcare workers. *J. Adv. Nurs.* **2008**, *62*, 84–95. [CrossRef]

66. Sane, M.A.; Devin, H.F.; Jafari, R.; Zohoorian, Z. Relationship between physical activity and it's components with burnout in academic members of Daregaz Universities. In *4th World Conference on Educational Sciences*; Baskan, G.A., Ozdamli, F., Kanbul, S., Ozcan, D., Eds.; Procedia—Social and Behavioral Sciences: Mashhad, Iran, 2012; Volume 46, pp. 4291–4294.

67. Jonsdottir, I.H.; Rödjer, L.; Hadzibajramovic, E.; Börjesson, M.; Ahlborg, G., Jr. A prospective study of leisure-time physical activity and mental health in Swedish health care workers and social insurance officers. *Prev. Med.* **2010**, *51*, 373–377. [CrossRef]

68. Lindwall, M.; Ljung, T.; Hadžibajramović, E.; Jonsdottir, I.H. Self-reported physical activity and aerobic fitness are differently related to mental health. *Ment. Health Phys. Act.* **2012**, *5*, 28–34. [CrossRef]

69. Gorter, R.C.; Eijkman, M.A.J.; Hoogstraten, J. Burnout and health among Dutch dentists. *Eur. J. Oral Sci.* **2000**, *108*, 261–267. [CrossRef]

70. Carson, N.E.; Blake, C.E.; Saunders, R. Perceptions and dietary intake of self-described healthy and unhealthy eaters with severe mental illness. *Community Ment. Health J.* **2015**, *51*, 281–288. [CrossRef]

71. Ekelund, U.; Steene-Johannessen, J.; Brown, W.J.; Fagerland, M.W.; Owen, N.; Powell, K.E.; Bauman, A.; Lee, I.M. Does physical activity attenuate, or even eliminate, the detrimental association of sitting time with mortality? A harmonised meta-analysis of data from more than 1 million men and women. *Lancet* **2016**, *388*, 1302–1310. [CrossRef]

72. Ciccone, J.; Woodruff, S.J.; Fryer, K.; Campbell, T.; Cole, M. Associations among evening snacking, screen time, weight status, and overall diet quality in young adolescents. *Appl. Physiol. Nutr. Metab.* **2013**, *38*, 789–794. [CrossRef]

73. Niermann, C.Y.N.; Spengler, S.; Gubbels, J.S. Physical Activity, Screen Time, and Dietary Intake in Families: A Cluster-Analysis with Mother-Father-Child Triads. *Front. Pub. Health* **2018**, *6*. [CrossRef]

74. Hall, K.D.; Heymsfield, S.B.; Kemnitz, J.W.; Klein, S.; Schoeller, D.A.; Speakman, J.R. Energy balance and its components: Implications for body weight regulation. *Am. J. Clin. Nutr.* **2012**, *95*, 989–994. [CrossRef]

75. Hill, J.O.; Wyatt, H.R.; Melanson, E.L. Genetic and environmental contributions to obesity. *Med Clin. North Am.* **2000**, *84*, 333–346. [CrossRef]

76. Armon, G.; Shirom, A.; Berliner, S.; Shapira, I.; Melamed, S. A prospective study of the association between obesity and burnout among apparently healthy men and women. *J. Occup. Heal. Psychol.* **2008**, *13*, 43–57. [CrossRef]

77. Piercy, K.L.; Troiano, R.P.; Ballard, R.M.; Carlson, S.A.; Fulton, J.E.; Galuska, D.A.; George, S.M.; Olson, R.D. The Physical Activity Guidelines for AmericansPhysical Activity Guidelines for AmericansPhysical Activity Guidelines for Americans. *JAMA* **2018**, *320*, 2020–2028. [CrossRef]

78. Cook, C.E.; George, S.Z.; Keefe, F. Different interventions, same outcomes? Here are four good reasons. *Br. J. Sports Med.* **2018**, *52*, 951–952. [CrossRef]

79. Grimby, G.; Borjesson, M.; Jonsdottir, I.H.; Schnohr, P.; Thelle, D.S.; Saltin, B. The "Saltin-Grimby Physical Activity Level Scale" and its application to health research. *Scand. J. Med. Sci. Sports* **2015**, *25* (Suppl. 4), 119–125. [CrossRef]

80. Tolkien, K.; Bradburn, S.; Murgatroyd, C. An anti-inflammatory diet as a potential intervention for depressive disorders: A systematic review and meta-analysis. *Clin. Nutr.* **2018**. [CrossRef]

81. Hagstromer, M.; Oja, P.; Sjostrom, M. The International Physical Activity Questionnaire (IPAQ): A study of concurrent and construct validity. *Public Health Nutr.* **2006**, *9*, 755–762. [CrossRef]

82. Maslach, C.; Jackson, S.; Leiter, M. *The Maslach Burnout Inventory Manual*; Consulting Psychologists Press: Palo Alto, CA, USA, 1997; Volume 3, pp. 191–218.

83. Chastin, S.F.M.; Schwarz, U.; Skelton, D.A. Development of a Consensus Taxonomy of Sedentary Behaviors (SIT): Report of Delphi Round 1. *PLoS ONE* **2013**, *8*. [CrossRef]

84. Kim, H.K.; Kim, M.J.; Park, C.G.; Kim, H.O. Gender differences in physical activity and its determinants in rural adults in Korea. *J. Clin. Nurs.* **2010**, *19*, 876–883. [CrossRef]

85. Azevedo, M.R.; Araújo, C.L.P.; Reichert, F.F.; Siqueira, F.V.; da Silva, M.C.; Hallal, P.C. Gender differences in leisure-time physical activity. *Int. J. Pub. health* **2007**, *52*, 8–15. [CrossRef]

86. Jones, F.; Harris, P.; Waller, H.; Coggins, A. Adherence to an exercise prescription scheme: The role of expectations, self-efficacy, stage of change and psychological well-being. *Br. J. Health Psychol.* **2005**, *10*, 359–378. [CrossRef]

87. Beer-Borst, S.; Hercberg, S.; Morabia, A.; Bernstein, M.S.; Galan, P.; Galasso, R.; Giampaoli, S.; McCrum, E.; Panico, S.; Preziosi, P.; et al. Dietary patterns in six european populations: Results from EURALIM, a collaborative European data harmonization and information campaign. *Eur. J. Clin. Nutr.* **2000**, *54*, 253–262. [CrossRef]

88. Wardle, J.; Haase, A.M.; Steptoe, A.; Nillapun, M.; Jonwutiwes, K.; Bellisle, F. Gender differences in food choice: The contribution of health beliefs and dieting. *Ann. Behav. Med.* **2004**, *27*, 107–116. [CrossRef]

89. Li, R.; Serdula, M.; Bland, S.; Mokdad, A.; Bowman, B.; Nelson, D. Trends in fruit and vegetable consumption among adults in 16 US states: Behavioral Risk Factor Surveillance System, 1990-1996. *Am. J. Public Health* **2000**, *90*, 777–781. [CrossRef]

90. Purvanova, R.; Muros, J. Gender differences in burnout: A meta-analysis. *J. Vocat. Behav.* **2010**, *77*, 168–185. [CrossRef]

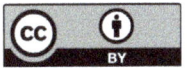

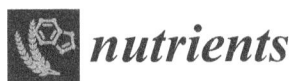

Review

Physical Activity in Eating Disorders: A Systematic Review

Rizk Melissa [1,2,3,*,†], **Mattar Lama** [4,†], **Kern Laurence** [5], **Berthoz Sylvie** [3,6], **Duclos Jeanne** [7,8], **Viltart Odile** [9,10] and **Godart Nathalie** [1,3]

[1] INSERM U1178, Maison de Solenn, 97 Boulevard De Port Royal, 75014 Paris, France; Nathalie.godart@fsef.net

[2] Université Paris-Sud and Université Paris Descartes, Ecole Doctorale des 3C (Cerveau, Cognition, Comportement), UMR-S0669, 75006 Paris, France

[3] Psychiatry Unit, Institut Mutualiste Montsouris 42, Boulevard Jourdan, 75014 Paris, France; Sylvie.berthoz-landron@inserm.fr

[4] Nutrition Program, Department of Natural Sciences, Lebanese American University, Beirut 1102, Lebanon; lama.mattar@lau.edu.lb

[5] Laboratoire EA 29 31, LINP2-APSA, et Laboratoire EA 4430 CLIPSYD Université Paris Nanterre UFR-STAPS, 200, Avenue de la République, 92001 Nanterre CEDEX, France; lkern@parisnanterre.fr

[6] INCIA UMR-5287 CNRS, Université de Bordeaux, 33076 Bordeaux, France

[7] Sciences Cognitives et Sciences Affectives, Université de Lille, CNRS, UMR 9193—SCALab, 59045 Lille, France; jeanne.duclos@univ-lille.fr

[8] Département de Psychiatrie, Hôpital Saint Vincent de Paul, GHICL, F-59000 Lille, France

[9] Institute of Psychiatry and Neurosciences of Paris, Unité Mixte de Recherche en Santé (UMRS) 1266 Institut National de la Santé et de la Recherche Médicale (INSERM), University Paris Descartes, 75014 Paris, France; odile.viltart@inserm.fr

[10] Department of Biology, University of Lille, 59000 Lille, France

* Correspondence: melissarizk@hotmail.com; Tel.: +33-787-483626

† Rizk Melissa and Mattar Lama contributed equally to the writing of this article.

Received: 27 November 2019; Accepted: 2 January 2020; Published: 9 January 2020

Abstract: Abnormally high levels of physical activity have been documented throughout the literature in patients with eating disorders (ED), especially those diagnosed with anorexia nervosa (AN). Yet no clear definition, conceptualization, or treatment of the problematic use of physical activity (PPA) in ED patients exists. The aim of this review is to propose a new classification of PPA, report the prevalence, triggers, predictors, maintainers and other related factors of PPA in ED patients, in addition to proposing a comprehensive model of the development of PPA in AN. A total of 47 articles, retrieved from Medline and Web of Science, met the inclusion criteria and were included in the analysis. As a result, the new approach of PPA was divided into two groups (group 1 and group 2) according to the dimension (quantitative vs qualitative approach) of physical activity that was evaluated. The prevalence of PPA in ED was reported in 20 out of 47 studies, the comparison of PPA between ED versus controls in 21 articles, and the links between PPA and psychological factors in ED in 26 articles, including depression (16/26), anxiety (13/26), obsessive–compulsiveness (9/26), self-esteem (4/26), addictiveness (1/26), regulation and verbal expression of emotions (1/26) and anhedonia (1/26). The links between PPA and ED symptomatology, PPA and weight, body mass index (BMI) and body composition in ED, PPA and age, onset, illness duration and lifetime activity status in ED, PPA and ED treatment outcome were reported in 18, 15, 7, 5 articles, respectively. All of the factors have been systematically clustered into group 1 and group 2. Results focused more on AN rather than BN due to the limited studies on the latter. Additionally, a model for the development of PPA in AN patients was proposed, encompassing five periods evolving into three clinical stages. Thus, two very opposite components of PPA in AN were suggested: voluntarily PPA increased in AN was viewed as a conscious strategy to maximize weight loss, while involuntarily PPA increased proportionally with weight-loss, indicating that exercise might be under the control of a subconscious biological drive and involuntary cognition.

Nutrients **2020**, *12*, 183

Keywords: review; eating disorders; physical activity; problematic use of physical activity

1. Introduction

A display of abnormally high levels of physical activity has been observed from the earliest clinical description of eating disorders (ED), especially in anorexia nervosa (AN) [1]. The latter has been considered to affect 31% to 80% of AN patients [2] and has been associated with a longer length of hospital stay [3], poor treatment outcome [4], interfering with refeeding strategies and body weight stabilization [5] and an increased risk of relapse and chronicity [6]. With more than 400 articles and seven partial reviews published on the subject in the past three decades, there is still no consensus on how to define, conceptualize or treat these observed high levels of physical activity in individuals suffering from ED. Physical activity is considered to be any body movement produced by the contraction of skeletal muscles, resulting in a substantial increase of energy expenditure relative to basal metabolism [7]. This has translated into a plethora of terms and definitions that has been described in social psychology by Hagger [8] who defines it as a "déjà-vu" phenomenon: "the feeling that one has seen a variable with the same definition and content before only referred to by a different term" [8] (p. 1). This might imply inconsistent or even contradictory findings, when in fact the definitions are the ambiguous factor [8]. In the current review, problematic use of physical activity in ED will be referred to as "problematic use of physical activity or PPA".

The seven previous reviews tackling the matter [2,9–14] did not adhere to the recommendation suggested by Hagger [15]. In other terms, they did not propose a redefinition/a model of the particular phenomena of PPA in ED. None of them considered all currently published studies, as some have been published earlier and/or have focused on only one aspect/dimension of the topic.

Researchers have given a plethora of terms and definitions to describe PPA in eating disorder patients [11]. Terms included "hyperactivity", "compulsive exercise", "driven exercise", "unhealthy exercise", "motor restlessness", "over-exercise", "overactivity", "hard exercise", "drive to exercise", "drive for activity", or "exercise dependence". This inconsistent use of terminology points out the ambiguity in defining this problematic behavior [16]. As mentioned by Adkins and Keel [17], definitions generally include a quantitative dimension of the behavior, including volume, frequency and/or intensity of exercise and/or a psychopathological dimension, while mentioning compulsivity and/or obsession and/or dependence to exercise. Multiple possible amalgamations can, therefore, be present and confuse the readers [15].

In light of the current gaps in the literature, the aims of this review are to:

– Propose a new classification of PPA based on the characteristics of physical activity and the nature of the relation that links the individual to his/her physical activity, independently of the name the authors had originally given it.
– Give an overview of the prevalence of PPA in ED patients; as well as the triggering, predicting, maintaining and other associated factors, using our proposed new classification of PPA, which takes into account the reported methodological discrepancies.
– Propose a comprehensive model of the development of PPA in AN.

2. Materials and Methods

A systematic literature search was performed according to the Preferred Reporting Items for Systematic Reviews and Meta-Analysis (PRISMA) statement [18].

2.1. Data Sources and Search Strategies

The information and relevant studies were retrieved by searching two on-line databases, MEDLINE and Web of Science. The following search strategy was conducted (adapted for each database): ("Eating disorders" OR "anorexia nervosa" OR "bulimia nervosa") AND ("Exercise" OR "physical activity"). Only articles in English or French, from all countries, published between the years 1970 and September 2019 (included) were reviewed. To identify further potentially relevant studies for inclusion, a complementary manual search of the titles, abstracts and reference lists of these articles was performed. When data were missing in the paper, additional information from study authors was systematically sought.

2.2. Study Selection

Eligible studies in the empirical literature should have aimed to evaluate the prevalence, the frequency, the nature and/or the clinical associated features (psychological or somatic) of physical activity in AN, Bulimia Nervosa (BN) and Eating Disorders Not Otherwise Specified (EDNOS). Our inclusion criteria limited our review to human studies that recruited all participants, or at least part of them, diagnosed with AN, BN with or without the mention of the subtypes; or EDNOS according to research diagnostic criteria. Thus, all studies on participants from the general population, athletes or animal models were excluded. Studies including other disorders such as Binge Eating Disorder or Attention Deficit Hyperactivity Disorder and case reports were excluded. All studies that did not match the aim of our review or papers on the treatment and/or management of physical activity in ED were not considered. The seven reviews mentioned in the introduction were also excluded as previously mentioned: none of them considered all currently published studies, as some are old and/or focused on only one aspect of the topic. Two independent reviewers (MR and NG) performed eligibility assessment individually. Disagreements between reviewers were resolved by consensus. Finally, 47 studies that met the inclusion criteria were identified and included in this paper. A flowchart summarizing the flow diagram of study selection is presented in Figure 1.

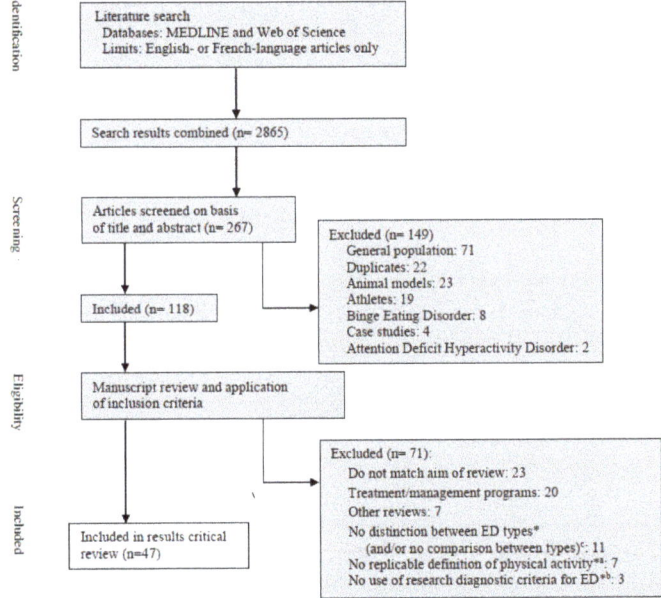

Figure 1. Flow diagram of the study selection. * Studies excluded for one or more reasons. [a] Blumenthal et al. (1984) [19]; Crisp et al. (1980) [20]; Davis et al. (1994) [21]; Frey et al. (2000) [22]; Kron et al. (1978) [23]; Monell et al. (2018) [24]; Sharp et al. (1994) [25]. [b] Blumenthal et al. (1984) [19]; Higgins et al. (2013) [26]; Long and Hollin (1995) [27]. [c] Boyd et al. (2007) [28]; Bratland-Sanda et al. (2010a, 2010b and 2011) [29–31]; Carruth and Skinner (2000) [32]; Davis et al. (1994 and 1998) [21,33]; Hechler et al. (2008) [34]; Naylor et al. (2011) [35]; Stiles-Shields et al. (2011) [36]; Vansteelandt et al. (2007) [37]. ED—eating disorders.

It was not possible to conduct a meta-analysis of the available studies due to the diversity of concepts and definitions used to evaluate PPA in ED.

3. Results

Aim number 1: Propose a new classification of PPA based on the characteristics of physical activity and the nature of the relation that links the individual to his/her physical activity, independently of the name the authors had originally given it.

Table 1 presents a plethora of terms and definitions used by authors, as well as the instruments used to assess PPA and the time of assessment.

We propose a new approach of PPA. It will categorize and differentiate the quantitative and the qualitative conceptualisations used in the literature, independently of the terms used by the authors, and divide studies into the following two groups:

- Group 1: Studies classified in this group determined PPA in a quantitative approach of physical activity in terms of intensity, frequency, duration and/or type of physical activity.
- Group 2: Studies classified in this group determined PPA in a qualitative approach by focusing on the relation that links an individual to his/her physical activity, including motives for exercise, compulsivity and exercise dependence/addiction, with or without a quantitative measure of physical activity.

Group 1 included 20 studies, group 2 included 20 studies, and seven studies were simultaneously in group 1 and group 2 (Table 2, column 2).

Table 1 summarizes terms used by authors, definitions, cut-offs, assessment instruments and time of assessment of PPA in ED. Results of study designs, diagnostic criteria of ED and sample composition are detailed in Table 3.

Aim number 2: Give an overview of the prevalence of PPA in ED patients and of the triggering, predicting, maintaining and other associated factors, using our proposed new classification of PPA, which takes into account the reported methodological discrepancies.

Table 1. Terms used by authors, definitions, cut-offs, assessment instruments and time of assessment of problematic use of physical activity in ED (columns 1 to 5).

1	2	3	4		5
			Assessment Instrument		
References Country	Terms Used by Authors	Definitions and Cut-Offs	Objectively	Subjectively	Time of Assessment
Falk et al. (1985) [38] USA	Energy expenditure/ motor activity	-	Actimetry	-	First 2 weeks of hospitalization.
Kaye et al. (1986) [39] USA	Physical activity	-	Acc.	-	3 to 5 day period of stable weight in hospital.
Casper et al. (1991) [40] USA	Energy expenditure	-	DLW	-	At time of admission to treatment program.
Pirke et al. (1991) [41] Germany	Hyperactivity and energy expenditure		DLW	PA diary	2 weeks after consenting to study (3 to 6 weeks in hospital).
Long et al. (1993) [12] Canada	Hyperactivity		-	1. ORQ 2. Modified CRQ (Carmack and Martens, 1979 [43])	First 2 weeks of hosp. in an ED unit.
Brewerton et al. (1995) [44] USA	Compulsive exercise	Exercise to control weight at least once a day and exercised for at least 60 min	-	DSED	-
Davis et al. (1995) [45] Canada	Excessive exercise	Exercise on average, a minimum of 5 h per week during the year prior to assessment	-	1. Interview 2. PA diary 3. CES	4 weeks and year prior to study inclusion.
Bouten et al. (1996) [46] The Netherlands	PA levels	Three PA levels: Low, moderate or high level.	1. Acc. 2. DLW	-	7 days after study inclusion.
Casper and Jabine (1996) [47] USA	Excessive exercise	Exercise more than 4 h per week of exercise for the month preceding the intake.	-	Interview	Month prior to hospitalization.
Davis et al. (1997) [48] Canada	Excessive exercise	Level of PA considerably more than typical for someone their age at that time and time spent exercising exceeded 1 h per day for at least 6 days per week for a period not less than 1 month, and if she described the exercising as "obsessive," "driven," and "out of control" during the excessive phase.	-	1. Interview 2. CES	Minimum 1 month prior to study inclusion.
Davis and Claridge (1998) [49] Canada	Excessive exercise	Lifetime exercise status: idem as Davis et al. (1997) [48]. Current exercise status: exercise activity for a minimum of 6 h a week averaged over the 12 months prior to assessment.	-	Interview	Year prior to study inclusion and during lifetime.
Davis et al. (1999) [50] Canada	Excessive exercise	Current exercise status: exercise activity for a minimum of 6 h a week averaged over 1 month prior to assessment.	-	1. Interview 2. CES	Minimum 1 month prior to study inclusion.
Favaro et al. (2000) [51] Italy	Excessive exercise	Excessive exercise as at least 1 h of intensive physical activity per day.	-	Interview	At start of outpatient treatment.
Pinkston et al. (2001) [52] USA	Energy expenditure	Three activity levels: Moderate, hard or very hard activities during the past 7 days.	-	1. 7d PAR 2. CES	At hospitalization.

Table 1. *Cont.*

References Country	Terms Used by Authors	Definitions and Cut-Offs	Assessment Instrument Objectively	Assessment Instrument Subjectively	Time of Assessment
Solenberger (2001) [3] USA	PA levels	"Patients were categorized into high- or low-level exercise groups by a median split of total exercise. The high-level exercise group spent greater than 6.7 h/week exercising".	-	Clinical charts	Six months prior to hospitalization.
Davis and Woodside (2002) [33] Canada	Excessive exercise	Exercise activity for a minimum of 6 h a week averaged over 1 month prior to assessment.	-	Interview	Minimum 1 month prior to study inclusion.
Penas-Lledo et al. (2002) [54] Spain	Excessive exercise	Physical exercise at least 5 times a week, for at least 1h without stopping, and with the aim of burning calories.	-	Clinical charts	-
Holtkamp et al. (2003) [55] Germany	Motor restlessness	Five levels of PA: no excessive physical activity; slight and/or rare excessive physical activity; marked and/or occasional excessive physical activity; strong and/or frequent excessive physical activity; very strong excessive physical activity.	-	SIAB-EX	3 months prior to hospitalization.
Holtkamp et al. (2004) [56] Germany	Excessive physical activity	Idem as Holtkamp et al. (2003) [55]	-	SIAB	3 months prior to hospitalization.
Klein et al. (2004) [57] USA	Exercise dependence	Exercise dependence if greater frequency of exercise ≥3 criteria of Modified SDSS	-	1. SDSS 2. CES	4 weeks prior to hospitalization.
Davis et al. (2005) [58] Canada	Excessive exercise	"Considerably more exercise/physical activity than is typical or normal for someone your age, and beyond the requirements of any competitive sport in which you were engaged".	-	1. Interview 2. CES	Year prior to hospitalization and lifetime.
Davis and Kaptein (2006) [59] Canada	Excessive exercise	Idem as Davis and Claridge (1998) [49] for lifetime and current exercise statuses.	-	Interview	Year prior to study inclusion and during lifetime.
Holtkamp et al. (2006) [60] Germany	PA levels and motor and inner restlessness	Idem as Holtkamp et al. (2003) [55]	Acc.	1. SIAB-EX 2. Self-report measures	3 months prior to hospitalization.
Shroff et al. (2006) [61] USA	Excessive exercise	Excessive exercise when any of the following were reported by the participant: (1) severe interference with important activities; (2) exercising more than 3 h/day and distress if unable to exercise; (3) frequent exercise at inappropriate times and places and little or no attempt to suppress the behavior; and (4) exercising despite more serious injury, illness or medical complication.	-	SIAB	3 months prior to hospitalization.
Klein et al. (2007) [62] USA	Excessive exercise	Exercising at least 6 h per week, on average.	Acc.	1. Interview 2. CES	3 months prior to hospitalization and during first 2 weeks of hospitalization.

Nutrients **2020**, 12, 183

Table 1. *Cont.*

References Country	Terms Used by Authors	Definitions and Cut-Offs	Assessment Instrument Objectively	Assessment Instrument Subjectively	Time of Assessment
Dalle Grave et al. (2008) [63] Italy	Compulsive exercise	Compulsive exerciser in the presence of a positive answer to the first question below and to anyone of the remaining: (1) Over the past 4 weeks, have you exercised with the aim of burning up calories to control your shape or weight? (2) Have you felt compelled or obliged to exercise? (3) Have you exercised even when it caused severe interference with important activities? (4) Have you exercised to a level that might be harmful for you? (5) Have you felt distressed if you were unable to exercise?	-	EDE	4 weeks prior to hospitalization.
Mond and Calogero (2009) [64] Australia	Excessive exercise	Exercise "hard as a means of controlling their shape or weight during the preceding 4 weeks".	-	1. EDE-Q 2. CES 3. REI	4 weeks prior to hospitalization.
Bewell-Weiss and Carter (2010) [65] Canada	Excessive exercise	Minimum of 1 h of obligatory exercise aimed at controlling shape and weight, 6 days per week in the month before admission.	-	EDE	3 months prior to hospitalization.
Thornton et al. (2011) [66] Sweden and USA	Excessive exercise	Exercise more than 2 h per day to control her shape and weight.	-	Interview	At time of interview.
Carrera et al. (2012) [67] The Netherlands	Physical activity levels/hyperactivity	Three PA intensities: Sedentary (<200 counts/min), light (200 to <1800 counts/min) and moderate to vigorous (≥1800 counts/min) activity.	Acc.	-	During 3 days after study inclusion.
Murray et al. (2012) [68] Australia	Compulsive exercise	-	-	CET	4 weeks prior to hospitalization.
Smith et al. (2012) [69] USA	Over-exercise	Exercise "hard as a means of controlling their shape or weight during the preceding 4 weeks".	-	EDE-Q	4 weeks prior to hospitalization.
El Ghoch et al. (2013) [70] Italy	PA energy expenditure	Two PA levels: light PA (<3 METs) and moderate and vigorous PA: (≥3 METs)	Acc.	-	During 1st week of hosp. and last week of day hospital.
Alberti et al. (2013) [71] Italy	PA energy expenditure	Three PA levels: Low PA (<3 METs), moderate PA (3 to 6 METs) and vigorous PA (>6 METs).	1. Acc. 2. IPAQ	-	At hospitalization.
Brownstone et al. (2013) [72] USA	Hard exercise	Exercise "hard as a means of controlling their shape or weight during the preceding 4 weeks".	-	EDE-Q	4 weeks prior to study inclusion.
Kostrzewa et al. (2013) [73] The Netherlands	PA levels and moderate-to-vigorous PA	Three levels of PA: Sedentary (<200 counts/min), light (200 to <1800 counts/min) and moderate-to-vigorous physical (≥1800 counts/min) activity.	Acc.	-	At hosp., end of hosp. and at 1 year follow-up.
Zipfel et al. (2013) [74] Australia	PA	From EDI-SC: "What percentage of your exercise is aimed at controlling your weight >50% cutoff"	DLW	1. DDE 2. EDI-SC	During hosp.

Table 1. *Cont.*

1	2	3	4 Assessment Instrument		5
References Country	Terms Used by Authors	Definitions and Cut-Offs	Objectively	Subjectively	Time of Assessment
Keyes et al. (2015) [75] United Kingdom	Drive to exercise	-	Actimetry	1. CES 2. OEQ GDES 3. EAI 4. IPAQ REI	During 7 days after study inclusion.
Sauchelli et al. (2015) [76] Spain	PA	Two PA levels: low exercisers (<300 min spent in moderate-to-vigorous PA) and high exercisers (≥300 min spent in moderate-to-vigorous PA).	Acc.	-	During 6 days after study inclusion.
Sternheim et al. (2015) [77] The Netherlands	Drive for activity	"urge to be physically active and an inability to sit still"	-	DFA-Q	At time of admission to treatment program.
Blachno et al. (2016) [78] Poland	PA	-	-	PAQ	Week prior to study inclusion.
El Ghoch et al. (2016) [79] Italy	PA energy expenditure	Two PA levels: light PA (<3 METs) and moderate and vigorous PA: (≥3 METs).	Acc.	-	During last week of day hospital.
Gianini et al. (2016) [80] USA	PA	-	Acc.	-	At hosp., at 90% weight gain in hospitalization and at 1 month after hospital discharge.
Noetel et al. (2016) [81] Australia	Compulsive exercise	-	-	CET	4 weeks prior to hospitalization.
Lehmann et al. (2018) [82] Germany	PA energy expenditure	Four PA levels: Very light-intensity PA ([1.1; 1.8] METs), light-intensity PA ([1.8; 3]), moderate-intensity PA ([3; 6] METs) and vigorous-intensity PA (≥6 METs).	Acc.	-	During hospitalization.
Schlegl et al. (2018) [83] Germany	Compulsive exercise	-	-	-CET -EMI-2	4 weeks prior to hospitalization.
Young et al. (2018) [84] Australia	Compulsive exercise	-	-	CET	4 weeks prior to hospitalization.

Acc.: Accelerometer. CEQ: Commitment to Exercise Questionnaire. CES: Commitment to Exercise Scale. CET: Compulsive Exercise Test. CRQ: Commitment to Running Questionnaire. DDE: Dieting Disorder Examination. DFA-Q: Drive for Activity Questionnaire. DLW: Double Labeled Water Method. DSED: Diagnostic Survey of the Eating Disorders. EAI: Exercise Addiction Inventory. EDE: Eating Disorder Examination. EDE-Q: Eating Disorder Examination Questionnaire. EDI-SC: Eating Disorders Inventory-Symptom Checklist. EDS-R: Exercise Dependence Scale—Revised. EEE-C: Eating and Exercise Examination-Computerized. EMA-Q: Ecological Momentary Assessment Questionnaire. EMI-2: Exercise Motivations Inventory-2. EPSQ: The Exercise Participation Screening Questionnaire. GAD: Generalized Anxiety Disorder. GDES: Global Drive to Exercise Score. IPAQ: International Physical Activity Questionnaire. MAQ: Modifiable Activity Questionnaire. METs: Metabolic equivalents [85]. ORQ: Obligatory Running Questionnaire. PA: Physical activity. PAQ: Physical activity questionnaire. PDPAR: Pediatric Physical Activity Recall. REI: Reasons for Exercise Inventory. SIAB: Structured Interview for Anorexic and Bulimic Disorders. SDSS: Substance Dependence Severity Scale. SIAB-EX: Structured Inventory for Anorexic and Bulimic Syndromes. 7d PAR: 7 days Physical Activity Recall. "-": no available data in study.

Table 2. Status and group classification of studies in the review and prevalence of problematic use of physical activity and statistical analysis used (columns 1 to 3).

1	2	3		
References Country	Group Classification	Prevalence (%)		
		AN	BN	Controls
Falk et al. (1985) [38] USA	Group 1	-	-	-
Kaye et al. (1986) [39] USA	Group 1	-	-	-
Casper et al. (1991) [40] USA	Group 1	-	-	-
Pirke et al. (1991) [41] Germany	Group 1	-	-	-
Long et al. (1993) [42] Canada	Group 2	-	-	-
Brewerton et al. (1995) [44] USA	Group 2 [b]	38.5	22.5	-
Davis et al. (1995) [45] Canada	Group 1 (Int.)	-	-	Sample 2: 37.5
	Group 2 (CES)			-
Bouten et al. (1996) [46] The Netherlands	Group 1	-	-	-
Casper and Jabine (1996) [47] USA	Group 1	75	-	-
Davis et al. (1997) [48] Canada	Group 2 [b]	80.8	57.1	-
Davis and Claridge (1998) [49] Canada	Group 1 (Current ex. st.)	47.08	32.65	-
	Group 2 (Lifetime ex. st.)	76.47	57.14	
Davis et al. (1999) [50] Canada	Group 1 (Current ex. st.)	69	-	-
	Group 2 (CES)	-		
Favaro et al. (2000) [51] Italy	Group 1	31.25	-	-
Pinkston et al. (2001) [52] USA	Group 1 (7d PAR)	-	-	-
	Group 2 (CES)			
Solenberger (2001) [3] USA	Group 1 [b]	54	39	-
Davis and Woodside (2002) [53] Canada	Group 1	-	-	-
Penas-Lledo et al. (2002) [54] Spain	Group 2	46	45.9	-
Holtkamp et al. (2003) [55] Germany	Group 2	-	-	-
Holtkamp et al. (2004) [56] Germany	Group 2	-	-	-
Klein et al. (2004) [57] USA	Group 2	48	-	-

Table 2. *Cont.*

1	2	3		
References **Country**	**Group** **Classification**	**Prevalence (%)**		
		AN	**BN**	**Controls**
Davis et al. (2005) [58] Canada	Group 1	64	-	2.1 *
Davis and Kaptein (2006) [59] Canada	Group 2	Current ex. st.: 50 Lifetime ex. st.: 80	-	-
Holtkamp et al. (2006) [60] Germany	Group 1 (acc.) Group 2 (SIAB)	-	-	-
Shroff et al. (2006) [61] USA	Group 2 [b]	ANR: 40.3 [a],*; ANP: 54.5 [a]; ANB: 37.4 [a],*; ANBN: 43.5 [a],*	BNP: 20.2 [a]; NPBN: 24 [a]	-
Klein et al. (2007) [62] USA	Group 1	41.7	-	-
Dalle Grave et al. (2008) [63] Italy	Group 2 [b]	AN-R: 80; AN-BP: 43.3	39.3	-
Mond and Calogero (2009) [64] Australia	Group 2 [b]	81.1	-	-
Bewell-Weiss and Carter (2010) [65] Canada	Group 2	34	-	-
Thornton et al. (2011) [66] Sweden and USA	Group 2	AN: 38.7; AN + GAD: 59.1	-	2.5
Carrera et al. (2012) [67] The Netherlands	Group 1	-	-	-
Murray et al. (2012) [68] Australia	Group 2	-	-	-
Smith et al. (2012) [69] USA	Group 2	-	-	-
Alberti et al. (2013) [71] Italy	Group 1	-	-	-
Brownstone et al. (2013) [72] USA	Group 2	-	204	-
El Ghoch et al. (2013) [70] Italy	Group 1	-	-	-
Kostrzewa et al. (2013) [73] The Netherlands	Group 1	30	-	-
Zipfel et al. (2013) [74] Australia	Group 2	58.3	-	16.7 *

Table 2. *Cont.*

1	2	3		
References Country	Group Classification	Prevalence (%)		
		AN	BN	Controls
Keyes et al. (2015) [75] United Kingdom	Group 1 (act.)	-	-	-
	Group 2 (GDES)			
Sauchelli et al. (2015) [76] Spain	Group 1	37.1	-	61.1
Sternheim et al. (2015) [77] The Netherlands	Group 2	-	-	-
Blachno et al. (2016) [78] Poland	Group 1	-	-	-
El Ghoch et al. (2016) [79] Italy	Group 1	-	-	-
Gianini et al. (2016) [80] USA	Group 1	-	-	-
Noetel et al. (2016) [81] Australia	Group 2	-	-	-
Lehmann et al. (2018) [82] Germany	Group 1	-	-	-
Schlegl et al. (2018) [83] Germany	Group 1 (Self-report)	-	-	-
	Group 2 (CET; EMI-2)			
Young et al. (2018) [84] Australia	Group 2	-	-	-

Acc.: Accelerometer. Act.: Actimetry. AN: Anorexia Nervosa. AN-R: Anorexia nervosa restricting-type. AN-BP: Anorexia nervosa binge-eating/purging type.BN: Bulimia Nervosa. CES: Commitment to Exercise Scale. CET: Compulsive Exercise Test. Current ex. st.: Current exercise status. EMI-2: Exercise Motivation Inventory-2. GAD: Generalized Anxiety Disorder. GDES: Global drive to exercise score. Int.: Interview. Lifetime ex. st.: Lifetime exercise status. Multi: Multivariate statistical analysis. SIAB: Structured Interview for Anorexic and Bulimic Disorders. Uni: Univariate statistical analysis. 7d PAR: 7 days Physical Activity Recall. "-": No available data in study. * $p < 0.05$. [a] According to Shroff and colleagues [61] unique form of categorization of lifetime ED subtypes: RAN: AN with restrictive eating and no purging or bingeing behavior; PAN: AN with purging behavior and no bingeing behavior; BAN: AN with bingeing with or without compensatory behaviors; PBN: BN with purging behavior; NPBN: BN with bingeing and no purging behavior. [b] Unfused samples (see "results" paragraph).

3.1. Prevalence of Problematic Use of Physical Activity in ED (20/47 Studies)

3.1.1. Problematic Use of Physical Activity in AN (20/20) and the Subtypes

In Group 1, the current prevalence of PPA varies from 30% to 75% according to the definitions or cut-off chosen (nine studies; Table 2, column 3).

Table 3. Methods of studies investigating problematic use of physical activity in ED (columns 1 to 11).

1	2	3	4	5	6	7	8	9	10	11
References Country	Study Design	Diagnostic Criteria	ED Subjects	Controls	Gender	Age (Years) Mean ± SD (Range)	Duration of Illness (Years) Mean ± SD (Range)	Age of Onset of ED (Years) Mean ± SD (Range)	Type of Treatment	Prevalence Period
Falk et al. (1985) [38] USA	Prospective case series	DSM-III	20 AN	-	Women	21.1 ± 5.6	-	-	In	Current
Kaye et al. (1986) [39] USA	Prospective case series	DSM-III	22 AN	11 healthy	Women	RW-R: 25.0 ± 1.1 LtW-R: 24.9 ± 1.7	RW-R = 84.1 ± 13.2 months LtW-R = 100.1 ± 14.7 months	RW-R = 17.6 ± 0.9 LtW-R = 16.5 ± 1.4	-	Lifetime 11 RW-R 11 LtW-R
Casper et al. (1991) [40] USA	Cross-sectional	DSM-III-R	6 AN	6 healthy	Women	24.5 ± 8	22.67 ± 10.7 months	-	Out	Current
Pirke et al. (1991) [41] Germany	Prospective case series	DSM-III-R	8 AN 8 BN	11 healthy	Women	AN: 27.8 ± 5.2 BN: 24.3 ± 4.7	-	-	In [d]	Current
Long et al. (1993) [42] Canada	Cross-sectional	DSM-III-R	21 AN	62 healthy	AN: women. Controls: 42 women; 20 men	25 ± 9.7	-	-	In	Current
Brewerton et al. (1995) [44] USA	Retrospective case series studies	DSM-III-R	18 AN 71 BN 21 EDNOS	-	Women	-	-	Ces: 12.1 ± 3.0 Non-Ces: 16.3 ± 1.8	In	Current
Davis et al. (1995) [45] Canada	Cross-sectional	DSM-III-R	46 AN	88 regular exercisers 40 high-level exercisers	Women	24.2 ± 4.7	-	-	In	Current
Bouten et al. (1996) [46] The Netherlands	Cross-sectional	DSM-III-R	11 AN	13 healthy	Women	33.6 ± 7.8	5 to 28	-	Out	Current
Casper and Jabine (1996) [47] USA	Follow-up	Feighner criteria	73 AN	-	Women	Early adolescent onset: 16.2 ± 3.3 Late adolescent onset: 19.7 ± 3.3 Adult onset: 25.2 ± 3.7	2.9	Early adolescent onset:13.9 ± 1.1 Late adolescent onset17.3 ± 0.8 Adult onset 22.2 ± 2.6	64 In 9 Out	Lifetime
Davis et al. (1997) [48] Canada	Cross-sectional	DSM-IV	Sample 1: 78 AN 49 BN; Sample 2: 40 AN	-	Women	Sample 1: 27.7 ± 7.8 Sample 2: 14.3 ± 1.5	-	-	In and Out	Current
Davis and Claridge (1998) [49] Canada	Cross-sectional	DSM-III-R	34 AN 49 BN	-	Women	28.1 ± 8.2	-	-	In and Out	Current and lifetime

Table 3. Cont.

1	2	3	4	5	6	7	8	9	10	11
References Country	Study Design	Diagnostic Criteria	ED Subjects	Controls	Gender	Age (Years) Mean ± SD (Range)	Duration of Illness (Years) Mean ± SD (Range)	Age of Onset of ED (Years) Mean ± SD (Range)	Type of Treatment	Prevalence Period
Davis et al. (1999) [50] Canada	Cross-sectional	DSM-IV	84 AN	-	Women	15.36 ± 1.38	11.6 ± 13.3 months	14.39 ± 1.38	In	Current
Favaro et al. (2000) [51] Italy	Cross-sectional	DSM-IV	13 AN-R 3 AN-BP	-	Women	22.3 ± 6.3	32.8 ± 43.4 months	-	Out	Current
Pinkston et al. (2001) [52] USA	Cross-sectional	DSM-III-R	11 EDNOS[a]	15 healthy	Women	20 ± 1.6	-	-	No treatment	Current
Solenberger (2001) [3] USA	Retrospective case series studies	DSM-IV-R	115 AN 38 BN 46 EDNOS		Women	20.6 ± 7.03	4.9 ± 0.49	-	In	Current
Davis and Woodside (2002) [53] Canada	Cross-sectional	DSM-IV	78 AN-R 76 BN 32 EDNOS	-	Women	27.0 ± 8.4	-	-	In and Out	Current
Penas-Lledo et al. (2002) [54] Spain	Retrospective case series	DSM-IV	35 AN-R 28 AN-BP 61 BN	-	Women	AN ex.: 18 ± 5.91 AN non-ex: 20.9 ± 6.38 BN ex: 20.1 ± 3.32 BN non-ex: 21.2 ± 4.72	-	-	Out	Current
Holtkamp et al. (2003) [55] Germany	Cross-sectional	DSM-IV	21 AN-R 6 AN-BP	-	Women	14.54 ± 1.299	-	-	In	Current
Holtkamp et al. (2004) [56] Germany	Cross-sectional	DSM-IV	23 AN-R 7 AN-BP	-	Women	14.6 ± 1	11 ± 7 months	-	In	Current
Klein et al. (2004) [57] USA	Cross-sectional	DSM-IV	8 AN-R 13 AN-BP	94 healthy	Women	23.38 ± 4.78	-	-	In	Current
Davis et al. (2005) [58] Canada	Cross-sectional	DSM-IV	125 AN-R 14 AN-BP		Women	15.3 ± 1.4	11.9 ± 1.2 months	14.3 ± 1.5	In	Current
Davis and Kaptein (2006) [59] Canada	Prospective case series	DSM-IV	50 AN-R	-	Women	25.4 ± 9.1	-	-	In	Current and lifetime
Holtkamp et al. (2006) [60] Germany	Cross-sectional	DSM-IV	26 AN	-	Women	15.6 ± 1.9	-	-	In	Current

Table 3. *Cont.*

1	2	3	4	5	6	7	8	9	10	11
References Country	Study Design	Diagnostic Criteria	ED Subjects	Controls	Gender	Age (Years) Mean ± SD (Range)	Duration of Illness (Years) Mean ± SD (Range)	Age of Onset of ED (Years) Mean ± SD (Range)	Type of Treatment	Prevalence Period
Shroff et al. (2006) [61] USA	Cross-sectional	DSM-IV	521 RAN c / 336 PAN c / 182 BAN c / 296 PBN c / 25 NPBN c / 400 ANBN / 96 EDNOS	-	Women	Ex: 26 ± 7.68 / Non-ex: 27.99 ± 9.51	Ex: 9.27 ± 6.93 / Non-ex: 9.41 ± 8.04	-	-	Lifetime
Klein et al. (2007) [62] USA	Cross-sectional	DSM-IV	14 AN-R / 22 AN-BP	-	Women	26.3 ± 5.9	-	-	In d	Current
Dalle Grave et al. (2008) [63] Italy	Prospective case series	DSM-IV	35 AN-R / 30 AN-BP / 28 BNP / 72 EDNOS	-	Women	26.0 ± 7.8	Ces: 94.3 ± 92.6 months / Non-Ces: 114.4 ± 92.3 months	AN: 16.5 ± 5.2 / BN: 17.9 ± 4.3 / EDNOS: 17.0 ± 6.0	In d	Current
Mond and Calogero (2009) [64] Australia	Cross-sectional	DSM-IV	15 AN-R / 13 AN-BP / 41 BN / 33 EDNOS	184 healthy	Women	AN-R: 21.0 ± 8.3 / AN-BP: 23.6 ± 8.3 / BN: 23.8 ± 6.2 / EDNOS: 20.5 ± 7.8	-	-	Out	Current
Bewell-Weiss and Carter (2010) [65] Canada	Cross-sectional	DSM-IV	98 AN-R / 61 AN-BP	-	148 women 5 men	26.0 ± 8.0	6.4 ± 8.0	-	In d	Current
Thornton et al. (2011) [66] Sweden and USA	Cross-sectional	DSM-IV	32 AN / 22 AN+GAD	5424 healthy	Women	AN: 34.8 ± 6 / AN+GAD: 30.1 ± 6.5	-	-	-	Lifetime
Carrera et al. (2012) [67] The Netherlands	Cross-sectional	DSM-IV	25 AN-R / 9 AN-BP / 3 EDNOS a	-	Women	15.3 ± 1.25	1.2 ± 0.79	-	5 In 32 Out	Current
Murray et al. (2012) [68] Australia	Cross-sectional	DSM-5	24 AN	15 gym-using	Men	23.92 ± 5.57	-	-	13 In 11 Out	Current
Smith et al. (2012) [69] USA	Cross-sectional	DSM-IV	144 BN / 60 EDNOS b	-	Women	25.67 ± 8.85	-	-	-	Current
Alberti et al. (2013) [71] Italy	Prospective case series	DSM-IV	52 AN	-	Women	24.4 ± 8.4	5 ± 9	-	In d	Current
Brownstone et al. (2013) [72] USA	Cross-sectional	DSM-IV	144 BN / 60 EDNOS b	-	Women	25.7 ± 8.8	-	-	-	Current

Table 3. *Cont.*

1	2	3	4	5	6	7	8	9	10	11
References Country	Study Design	Diagnostic Criteria	ED Subjects	Controls	Gender	Age (Years) Mean ± SD (Range)	Duration of Illness (Years) Mean ± SD (Range)	Age of Onset of ED (Years) Mean ± SD (Range)	Type of Treatment	Prevalence Period
Kostrzewa et al. (2013) [73] The Netherlands	Prospective case series and follow-up	DSM-IV	25 AN-R, 9 AN-BP, 3 EDNOS^a	-	Women	15.15 ± 1.21	-	-	23 In, 14 Out^d	Current
Zipfel et al. (2013) [74] Australia	Prospective case series	DSM-IV	8 AN-R, 4 AN-BP	12 healthy	Women	21.9 ± 6.2	4.3 ± 3.9	-	In^d	Current
Keyes et al. (2015) [75] United Kingdom	Prospective case series	DSM-IV	55 AN	30 healthy, 34 anxiety	Women	29	-	-	18 In, 37 Out	Current
Sauchelli et al. (2015) [76] Spain	Prospective case series	DSM-IVTR	52 AN-R, 36 AN-BP	116 healthy	Women	27.94 ± 9	7.2 ± 6.4	21.2 ± 8.4	In^d	Current
Sternheim et al. (2015) [77] The Netherlands	Cross-sectional	DSM-5	145 AN-R, 95 AN-BP	-	Women	21.6 ± 8.9	5.5 ± 7.4	15.7 ± 4.0	Out	Current
Blachno et al. (2016) [78] Poland	Prospective case series	DSM-IV and ICD-10	76 AN	-	Women	14.8 ± 1.8	-	-	In	Current
El Ghoch et al. (2016) [79] Italy	Prospective case series and follow-up	DSM-IV	32 AN	-	Women	22.45	-	-	In^d	Current
Gianini et al. (2016) [80] USA	Prospective case series and follow-up	DSM-5	61 AN	24 healthy	Women	24.4 ± 6.5	8.3 ± 6.6	-	In	Current
Noetel et al. (2016) [81] Australia	Prospective case series	DSM-5	60 AN	-	Women	15.02 ± 1.22	1.12 ± 0.98	-	In^d	Current
Lehmann et al. (2018) [82] Germany	Prospective case series	ICD-10	24 AN-R, 13 AN-BP, 13 AN atypical	30 healthy	Women	25	6.25	-	In	Current
Schlegl et al. (2018) [83] Germany	Prospective case series	ICD-10	151 AN, 75 BN	109 healthy	Women	AN: 21.11 ± 6.94; BN: 23.09 ± 7.6	-	-	In	Current
Young et al. (2018) [84] Australia	Cross-sectional	DSM-5	56 AN-R, 22 AN-BP	-	74 women, 4 men	27.38 ± 9.22	5.65 ± 7.88	-	Out	Current

AN: Anorexia Nervosa. BN: Bulimia nervosa. DSM: Diagnostic Statistical Manual. EDNOS: Eating disorder not otherwise specified. ED: Eating disorder. AN-R: Anorexia nervosa restricting-type. AN-BP: Anorexia nervosa binge-eating/purging type. AN-BN: lifetime diagnosis of AN and BN. BN-P: Bulimia nervosa purging type. RW-R: Recently weight-recovered; LtW-R: long-term weight-recovered; Ex: Excessive exercisers. Ces: Compulsive exercisers. GAD: Generalized Anxiety Disorder. In: Inpatient treatment. Out: Outpatient treatment. Day: Day treatment. "-": no available data in study. ^a EDNOS patients that were considered AN in review. See review part II. ^b EDNOS patients that were considered BN in review. See review part II. ^c According to Shroff and colleagues [61] unique form of categorization of lifetime ED subtypes: RAN: AN with restrictive eating and no purging or bingeing behavior; PAN: AN with purging behavior and no bingeing behavior; BAN: AN with bingeing with or without compensatory behaviors; PBN: BN with purging behavior; NPBN: BN with bingeing and no purging behavior. ^d Study that gave details about ED treatment program.

In Group 2, we found 14 prevalence for PPA in 12 studies. Lifetime prevalence were given by four studies [49,59,61,66]. Current prevalence varied from 34% to 58% (Table 2, column 3). The two with the largest sample size [63,65] were both in favor of higher PPA in AN-R patients compared to AN-BP. Klein et al. [57], who compared only 8 AN-R with 13 AN-BP patients, failed to find a significant difference.

Shroff et al. [61], who described lifetime ED subtypes (usually diagnosed transversely) found significantly higher PPA in ANP (according to their own categorization, cf. Table 3 for details of categorization) than all other subtypes of AN including, what they called, restrictive AN and BN participants and individuals with a lifetime diagnosis of AN and BN.

3.1.2. Problematic Use of Physical Activity in BN (9/20)

Among BN patients, both prevalence of PPA in Groups 1 and 2 seemed to be strongly affected by the way they were defined and measured. There were no studies comparing BN patients to healthy controls.

In Group 1 (2/9), PPA varies between 32.6% and 39% in two studies [3,49] (Table 2, column 4).

In Group 2 (1/9), regarding lifetime prevalence, the only study available reported 57% of PPA in BN [48]. Five studies considered current BN status and reported the prevalence of PPA as varying from 20.2% (either current or past ED; [61]) to 60% [69].

3.1.3. Comparison of Problematic Use of Physical Activity between AN and BN (10/20)

In the studies comparing PPA in AN and BN [3,41,44,48,49,54,61,63,64,83], AN were found to be physically more active than BN in: (a) Group 1, four studies [3,41,61,83] out of five [49] found no significant difference for current exercise status. (b) Group 2, three out of six studies [44,48,63] while the three others found no significant difference [49] (only for lifetime exercise status) [54,83].

3.2. *Comparison of Problematic Use of Physical Activity between ED Versus Controls (21/47)*

3.2.1. Problematic Use of Physical Activity in AN Patients Versus Controls (21/21)

Prevalence of PPA in Group 1 was investigated in two studies [58,76], and the results were contradictive. Davis et al. [58] found significantly more excessive exercisers among the AN patients than among healthy controls. However, physical activity was significantly higher in healthy controls compared to AN inpatients [76].

Energy expenditure was measured in six studies [40,41,52,70,75,80] and exercise duration in one study [83]. Energy expended during physical activity [40,70] and duration of exercise [83] were significantly higher in AN patients compared to control subjects.

3.2.2. Problematic Use of Physical Activity in BN Patients Versus Controls (2/21)

In Group 1, no significant group differences were found both in energy expenditure (in kilo calories per day) [41], nor in the duration of physical activity (in minutes per day) [41,83].

In Group 2, BN patients scored higher on the CET's rule-driven behaviour, weight control exercise, mood improvement and exercise rigidity subscales than healthy controls [83].

3.3. *Links between Problematic Use of Physical Activity and Comorbidities and Psychological Factors in ED (26/47)*

The comorbidities and psychological factors that have been investigated in ED patients will be reviewed below in the following order: depression (16/26), anxiety (13/26), obsessive–compulsiveness (9/26), self-esteem (4/26), addictiveness (1/26), regulation and verbal expression of emotions (1/26) and anhedonia (1/26) (Table 4). When BN is not mentioned, the latter implies absence or non-significant data.

Table 4. Instruments used to assess comorbidities, psychological factors, and ED symptomatology (Columns 1 to 4).

1 References Country	2 Group Classification	3 Depression	Anxiety	Ob-Co	Self-Esteem	Stress	Addict.	Regul.	Anhedonia	4 ED Symptomatology
Falk et al. (1985) [38] USA	Group 1	HRS	-	-	-	-	-	-	-	-
Casper et al. (1991) [40] USA	Group 1	BDI	-	-	-	-	-	-	-	EDI; EAT
Long et al. (1993) [42] Canada	Group 2	BSI	BSI	-	SEI	-	-	-	-	EAT; EDI
Davis et al. (1995) [45] Canada	Groups 1 and 2	-	-	SCL-90	-	-	-	-	-	EDI
Casper and Jabine (1996) [47] USA	Group 1	-	-	-	GAS	-	-	-	-	-
Davis et al. (1997) [48] Canada	Group 2	-	-	-	-	-	-	-	-	Self-report psychological inventories
Davis et al. (1999) [50] Canada	Groups 1 and 2	-	-	Lazare et al. Inventory *	-	-	EPQ-R	-	-	-
Favaro et al. (2000) [51] Italy	Group 1	HSCL	HSCL	-	-	-	-	-	-	EDI; 24-h dietary recalls; 3-day food record
Davis and Woodside (2002) [53] Canada	Group 1	SCL-90	-	-	-	-	-	-	Physical Anhedonia scale	-
Penas-Lledo et al. (2002) [54] Spain	Group 2	SCL-90-R	SCL-90-R	SCL-90-R	-	-	-	-	-	EAT-40; BITE
Holtkamp et al. (2004) [56] Germany	Group 2	SCL-90-R	SCL-90-R	SCL-90-R	-	-	-	-	-	SIAB
Klein et al. (2004) [57] USA	Group 2	BDI	BAI	-	-	-	-	-	-	YBC-EDS
Davis et al. (2005) [58] Canada	Group 1	-	-	-	-	-	-	-	-	EDI; Interview
Davis and Kaptein (2006) [59] Canada	Group 2	-	-	MOCI; Lazare et al. Inventory *	-	-	-	-	-	-
Klein et al. (2007) [62] USA	Group 1	BDI	BAI	-	-	-	-	-	-	EDI
Bewell-Weiss and Carter (2010) [65] Canada	Group 2	BDI-2	BSI	Padua Inventory	Rosenberg Self-Esteem Scale	-	-	-	-	EDE-Q; EDI
Thornton et al. (2011) [66] Sweden and USA	Group 2	-	GAD	-	-	-	-	-	-	-

Table 4. Cont.

References Country	Group Classification	Depression	Anxiety	Ob-Co	Self-Esteem	Stress	Addict.	Regul.	Anhedonia	ED Symptomatology
					Comorbidities and Psychological Factors					
Carrera et al. (2012) [67] The Netherlands	Group 1	CDI	STAI	-	-	-	-	-	-	EDI-2
Brownstone et al. (2013) [72] USA	Group 2	-	-	-	-	-	-	DAPP-BQ	-	EDE-Q
Kostrzewa et al. (2013) [73] The Netherlands	Group 1	CPRS-S-A	CPRS-S-A	CPRS-S-A	-	-	-	-	-	EDI-2; MROAS
Zipfel et al. (2013) [74] Australia	Group 2	BDI	-	-	-	-	-	-	-	EAT; EDI-2
Keyes et al. (2015) [75] United Kingdom	Groups 1 and 2	DASS	DASS	-	-	DASS	-	-	-	EDE-Q
Sauchelli et al. (2015) [76] Spain	Group 1	SCL-90-R	-	-	-	-	-	-	-	EDI-2
Sternheim et al. (2015) [77] The Netherlands	Group 2	-	STAI	-	-	-	-	-	-	EDE
Blachno et al. (2016) [78] Poland	Group 1	-	-	LOI-CV	-	-	-	-	-	-
Noetel et al. (2016) [81] Australia	Group 2	RCADS	RCADS	ChOCI-R	Rosenberg Self-Esteem Scale	-	-	-	-	Y-EDEQ

Addict.: Addictiveness. ED: Eating disorders. BAI: Beck Anxiety Inventory. BSI: Brief Symptom Inventory. BITE: Bulimic Investigatory Test, Edinburg. ChOCI-R: Children's Obsessional Compulsive Inventory-Revised. CPRS-S-A: Comprehensive Psychopathological Rating Scale. DAPP-BQ: Dimensional Assessment of Personality Pathology - Basic Questionnaire. DASS: Depression Anxiety Stress Scale 21-version. EAT: Eating Attitudes Test. EDE-Q: Eating Disorder Examination–Self-Report Questionnaire Version. EDI: Eating Disorder Inventory. EPQ-R: Eysenck Personality Questionnaire-Revised. GAD diagnosis: Generalized anxiety disorder diagnosis. GAS: Global Assessment Scale. HRS: Hamilton Rating Scale. HSCL: Hopkins Symptom Checklist. LOI-CV: Leyton Obsessional Inventory–Child Version. MMPI: Minnesota Multiphasic Personality Inventory. MOCI: Maudsley Obsessive–Compulsive Inventory. MROAS: Morgan and Russell Outcome Assessment Schedule. Ob-Co: Obsessive–Compulsiveness. RCADS: Revised Child Anxiety and Depression Scale. Regul.: Regulation and verbal expression of emotions. SCID: Structured Clinical Interview for DSM-IV. SCL-90: Symptom Check-List-90. SCL-90-R: Symptom Check-List-90-Revised. SEI: Culture Free Self Esteem Inventory. SIAB: Structured Interview of Anorexia and Bulimia Nervosa. STAI: State-Trait Anxiety Inventory. YBC-EDS: Yale-Brown-Cornell Eating Disorder Scale. Y-EDEQ: Youth Eating Disorder Examination-Questionnaire. "-": No available data in study; * Inventory designed to assess the "obsessional" or "anal" personality type derived from psychoanalytic theory [86,87].

3.3.1. Depression in AN

Group 1 included six studies and the majority of them (5/6) did not find any association between PPA and depression [62,67,73,75,76]. Only Falk et Al. [38], found that patients that were less active at admission were also more depressed, but this association disappeared after 14 days of hospitalization.

Group 2 included eight studies: five [54,56,65,74,75] reported a positive proportional association between depression, on both categorical and dimensional approaches, and exercise status, including frequency and volume of exercise. Furthermore, Zipfel et al. [74] found that the patient's level of depressive symptoms was positively correlated to total daily energy expenditure. In addition, out of the four studies that found no association between depression and PPA, Long et al. [42] found nonetheless that depression was associated with a greater tendency for secret and solitary exercising in anorexics. The two remaining studies were those with the smallest samples ($n = 30$ and $n = 21$) [56,57].

3.3.2. Anxiety in AN

Group 1 included four studies [62,67,73,75], which all failed to find an effect of anxiety: (a) when comparing high/non-high exercisers [62,73]; (b) using correlations between the level of anxiety and general physical activity measured in counts/day by an accelerometer [67] or actimetry [75]; (c) when comparing two levels of physical activity that are sedentary and light physical activity [67]. However, Carrera et al. [67] noticed that the more time AN patients spent in the moderate to vigorous physical activity level, the less they reported to be anxious (cf. Table 4).

Group 2 included nine studies. All studies except one [65] found an increase in PPA in cases of elevated anxiety.

Furthermore, Long et al. [42] found that anxiety levels and phobic anxiety were associated with a greater tendency for solitary and secret exercising in AN. They also found that individuals suffering from AN were more likely to cope with negative emotional states (referring to feelings of anxiety, anger, low mood/depression) by using exercise than normal controls.

In addition, Penas-Lledo et al. [54] found that AN patients who exercised had significantly greater levels of somatization in addition to anxiety than the ones who did not exercise. Thornton et al. [66] found that significantly more individuals suffering from AN with or without generalized anxiety disorder (GAD) reported more PPA than healthy controls and women with GAD only.

3.3.3. Obsessive–Compulsiveness in AN

Group 1 included only two studies [73,78], which did not find a significant difference between excessive and non-excessive exercisers. However, Blachno et al. [78] found that adolescent patients at high risk of obsessive–compulsive disorder reported more intentional physical activities aimed at weight loss than the non-high-risk group.

Group 2 included seven studies: Obsessive–compulsiveness was found to be associated with PPA in three of these studies [45,50,59,81], with pathologically motivated exercisers reporting more obsessive–compulsive personality characteristics and greater obsessional-compulsive disorder symptoms than non-pathologically motivated exercisers [59]. Surprisingly, Bewell-Weiss and Carter [65], who used a totally different instrument (Padua Inventory, [88]) found that obsessive–compulsiveness was negatively associated with PPA in AN. The remaining two studies [54,56] found no association between obsessive–compulsiveness and PPA. No statistical association was found between obsessive–compulsive traits and addictive personality in childhood and adolescent activity levels of AN patients [50].

3.3.4. Self-Esteem and Addictiveness in AN

Self-esteem was found to be positively associated with PPA in patients suffering from AN in Group 2 [65,81]. The study by Davis et al. [50], which is also classified into Group 2, found that an addictive personality in AN significantly predicted the degree to which patients reported obligatory attitudes to exercising. There were no data in the literature regarding BN patients.

3.3.5. Regulation and Verbal Expression of Emotions in BN

A study by Brownstone et al. [72], classified into Group 2, found that only BN patients with high levels of compulsivity engaged in more PPA when they presented high levels of affect lability compared to low levels of affect lability. They found a trend for the same association in the case of high compulsivity's association between PPA and restricted emotion.

3.3.6. Anhedonia in ED

The study by Davis and Woodside [53], which can be classified into Group 1, found that exercise status, i.e., excessive vs. non-excessive exercisers, contributed positively to the variance in the level of anhedonia reported by patients with AN, independently of patient differences in depression severity. They also found that BN patients belonging to the non-excessive exercise group had significantly lower anhedonia scores than both BN patients in the excessive exercise group and AN patients belonging to the non-excessive exerciser group.

3.4. Links between Problematic Use of Physical Activity and ED Symptomatology in AN (18/47)

ED symptomatology was studied either globally or focused on one aspect, such as weight preoccupation, drive for thinness, body dissatisfaction or eating behaviors.

Group 1 included eight studies. Three examined general eating disorder pathology and found no association with either locomotor activity [62], actimetry [75], or levels of physical activity [73,76]. When taking into account peak activity (highest per minute level of activity in a 5 min period), PPA was correlated to EDE-Q higher scores [75].

However, significant associations were reported when the core ED symptoms were studied separately. In fact, Davis et al. [45] found that weight preoccupation was positively related to AN patients' level of physical activity. Two studies [40,51] focused on comparing ED symptoms between AN patients and healthy controls and found that PPA in AN patients was significantly associated with greater body dissatisfaction and drive for thinness than controls. Nevertheless, Carrera et al. [67] found that body dissatisfaction subscale scores of the Eating Disorders Inventory (2nd version) were not a significant predictor of PPA in AN.

Group 2 included seven studies with mainly the following results: (1) Weight preoccupation was found positively related to PPA among AN patients [58]; (2) Greater levels of general eating symptoms and bulimic scores were found in AN outpatients who exercised than in those who did not [54]; (3) Drive for thinness was found to be positively associated with PPA in AN [74]; (4) Quantitative food restriction was found to be positively related to PPA in AN patients, even when anxiety was taken into account [56]; (5). PPA was positively correlated with general eating pathology scores of AN outpatients [75,77] and AN inpatients [81]. In fact, Keyes et al. [75] found that ED pathology, along with exercising to improve mood, contributed the most to the variance in PPA in these patients (25.3% and 26.5%, respectively).

3.5. Links between Problematic Use of Physical Activity and Weight, Body Mass Index (BMI) and Body Composition in ED (15/47)

Five studies used bioelectrical impedance to assess body composition in their study samples, [40,41,73,76,82]; yet none used a validated equation for ED population [89]. Given the differences in instruments used to measure PPA, very heterogeneous results were observed.

3.5.1. Weight, BMI and Body Composition in AN (12/12)

Group 1 included 11 studies [38,40,41,46,57,67,73,76,79,80,82]. Four studies failed to find a significant difference between excessive and non-excessive exercisers or physical activity levels with regard to body mass index (BMI) [41,57,67,73,80] and body composition [41,73]. Other studies found that body weight [38,82], BMI [40,46,76,82], resumption of menses [70] and percentage of body fat [40,82] were positively related to the level of daily physical activity. Moreover, Bouten et al. [46] found that the intensity of physical activity (in counts per minute, measured by an accelerometer) in AN outpatients increased significantly with BMI values ≥ 15 kg·m^{-2}. Below this value, physical activity was assumed to reach a minimum.

Group 2 included four studies with different results. Two studies [56,77] found that BMI was not significantly correlated to PPA. However, Keyes et al. [75] found that PPA was negatively correlated to BMI. Penas-Lledo et al. [54], in a clinical chart analysis, found that AN patients who reported PPA had higher BMIs than the ones who did not.

3.5.2. Weight, BMI and Body Composition in BN (2/11)

In Group 1, Pirke et al. [41] found no association between PPA, BMI or body composition. In Group 2, Penas-Lledo et al. [54] found that BN patients who reported PPA had higher BMIs than non-exercisers.

3.6. *Links between Problematic Use of Physical Activity, Age, Onset, Illness Duration, Quality of Life and Lifetime Activity Status in ED (7/49)*

3.6.1. Age, Onset, Illness Duration and Lifetime Activity Status in AN (7/7)

Group 1 included five studies. The link between patient's age and PPA was examined in three studies, with concordant results. None of the studies found an association between AN inpatient's age and their level of locomotor activity [62] or of physical activity [67,73].

Davis et al. [58] measured physical activity levels during childhood and found an increase of the level of physical activity with age for both AN patients and controls; however, a greater rate was observed for AN patients. In addition, a large change in the amount of physical activity approximately one year prior to the onset of AN was detected.

Moreover, Davis et al. [48] found that AN patients who exercise excessively had a significant increase in physical activity levels around one year prior to the onset of the disease. An earlier age of onset of AN was associated with both quantitative and qualitative dimensions of PPA [48,73].

Finally, Kostrzewa et al. [73] found that, before admission to treatment, AN excessive exercisers had longer illness duration than the non-excessive exercisers group.

Group 2 included three studies that measured lifetime PPA status among AN adolescents. Davis et al. [48] found that the currently "more active" patients were also more involved in sport and exercise activities at ages 10 and 12 than their less-active counterparts. Davis et al. [50] found that a greater number of patients who had been highly active as children subsequently engaged in more PPA during their illness than those who were average/less active as children. However, Noetel et al. [81] failed to find an association between PPA and duration of illness in their adolescent sample.

3.6.2. Age, Onset, Illness Duration and Lifetime Activity Status in BN (1/7)

The study by Davis et al. [48], which can be classified into Group 2, found that a greater proportion of BN adult patients started dieting before starting to regularly exercise (or dieted without ever exercising) than the ones who started exercising before reducing their food consumption.

3.6.3. Quality of Life (2/7)

Quality of life has been found to be negatively impacted by the effect of PPA (in Group 2) interacting with ED severity [84,90].

3.7. Links between Problematic Use of Physical Activity and ED Treatment Outcome (5/49)

3.7.1. ED Treatment Outcome in AN (4/5)

Group 1 included five studies. Kostrzewa et al. [73] found that recovery, defined as having a score equal or superior to nine on the Morgan and Russell outcome assessment schedule, was predicted by significantly higher physical activity levels at inclusion. They also found a decrease in activity levels for excessive exercisers at one year of follow-up; however, the activity levels stabilized after that. However, Lehmann et al. [82] did not find intensity and duration of physical activity to be significant predictors of percentage of BMI increase between admission and discharge to an inpatient treatment. Gianini et al. [80] found total physical activity to be higher in patients at a weight restoration of 90% in an inpatient treatment compared to the start of hospitalization.

El Ghoch et al. [70] studied treatment dropouts and their results were twofold: (1) They found a positive association between PPA and treatment dropout in AN inpatients, with dropouts having higher moderate and vigorous physical activity duration and expenditure at baseline than completers. They failed to find an association between end-of-treatment physical activity assessment measures ED or general psychiatry features between AN completers vs. dropouts. They also failed to find a significant difference in EE assessment when comparing AN subtypes of patients who completed their treatment with those who did not. (2). For the comparison between AN patients who completed their treatment with healthy controls, AN completers were found to have a higher number of daily steps, duration and moderate–vigorous physical activity expenditure. Kostrzewa et al. [73] did not confirm this result in their adolescent (and smaller) sample.

El Ghoch et al. [79] found that the number of daily steps at inpatient discharge was the only independent predictor of menstrual resumption; the non-menstruating inpatient group performed a higher number of daily steps than the menstruating group at discharge.

3.7.2. ED Treatment Outcome in BN (1/5)

A study by Smith et al. [69], which can be included in Group 2, were the only ones to examine, in a sample of adult suffering from BN, the links between PPA and suicide in a multivariate analysis. Smith et al. [69] found that PPA was positively associated with suicidal gestures and attempts even when controlling for frequency of vomiting episodes, laxative abuse, dietary restraint and age.

4. Discussion

We hypothesized that categorizing studies into two groups would lead to a harmonization of their results and make a comparison between them possible (cf. results aim 1). This was only partially verified. Indeed, the classification we proposed did not decrease the wide range of prevalence generally given in the literature of 31% to 80% [2]. Our group classification showed that a high level of PPA (group 2) is associated with more anxiety, obsessive–compulsiveness and addictiveness, and higher self-esteem, which was not the case for studies using PPA evaluations (group 1). We were also able to confirm that AN patients have more PPA than healthy controls independently of the quantitative or qualitative dimension studied.

4.1. Prevalence of Problematic Use of Physical Activity

The ranges of prevalence in both cases are inarguably highly dependent on: (1) the cut-off used by authors to divide their study sample into high vs. low exercisers, sometimes doubling from one study to another; (2) the sample composition (inpatients vs. outpatients and AN vs. BN); (3) evaluation methods (subjective vs. objective measures). Indeed, current prevalence was considered during hospitalization, which directly or indirectly limits PPA [5]. Furthermore, methods of self-evaluation are highly critical among AN patients who are known to hide/underestimate (considering self-reports) their symptoms [91].

In addition, an important factor affecting PPA prevalence was that lifetime PPA was nearly two-times higher than the current prevalence (80% vs. 46%); therefore, we considered those data separately.

4.2. Comparison of Problematic Use of Physical Activity between ED Patients Versus Controls

Compared to healthy controls, AN patients had higher frequencies of PPA if PA was measured subjectively. Objectively, healthy controls were found to be more physically active than AN inpatients [76]. This is not surprising since, as mentioned previously, hospitalized patients have limited PA.

A lack of research devoted to AN patients that have low to no physical activity levels in comparison with those having high PPA was observed. We are compelled to think that they could (1) have low BMI since Bouten et al. [46] found that physical activity reached a minimum at BMI values below $15 \text{ kg} \cdot \text{m}^{-2}$; and/or (2) be more depressed, as Falk et al. [38]; and/or (3) more frequently classified as AN binge–purging type [44].

At least partially against this view, Davis [9] discussed that AN patients feel an increasingly strong compulsion to be physically active, despite pain and exhaustion. No studies focus on the question of the threshold of nutritional statuses that lead to a decrease in PPA, nor if this absence of adaptive and progressive decrease in PPA, linked to exhaustion, could define a subgroup of AN patients, observed clinically. This subgroup is the one that could have PPA until death.

4.3. Problematic Use of Physical Activity, Comorbidities and Psychological Factors

Since depression, anxiety and obsessive–compulsive disorder frequently co-occur with AN [92–94], it was not surprising to find that they were the most studied psychological factors to be linked together with ED and PPA. We can see here all the interest of using our classification to re-analyze inconclusive results found in previous reviews, with results from Group 1 frequently being the opposite than Group 2.

PPA only considered quantitatively (Group 1) was found to be negatively correlated to depression [38] or completely not associated to it. This was also the case in the general population, where greater amounts of occupational and leisure time activities, as well as all physical activity intensity levels, were generally associated with reduced symptoms of depression [95,96], anxiety and stress [38].

However, when focusing on PPA (group 2) and thus taking into account the pathological motivations linked to ED, we observed the opposite effect: depression (or depressive disorder), anxiety, obsessive–compulsiveness, addictiveness, and higher self-esteem were significantly positively associated with PPA. The more an AN patient has those symptoms, the more he/she practiced PPA. This could be explained by the fact patients were trying to improve their mood and emotional state [9,42,54,75,83] with physical activity being considered as a way of coping with a chronically negative affect [37] by pursuing the boosting effect of endogenous opioids [10].

4.4. Problematic Use of Physical Activity and ED Symptomatology

Keyes et al. [75] found that ED pathology was one of the most important predictors of the variance of PPA in Group 2 in AN outpatients, but when compared to healthy controls, PPA in AN patients were significantly and positively associated with drive for thinness. It seems that AN patients are likely to increase their levels of PPA (quantitatively and qualitatively) when preoccupied about their weight and motivated by their drive for thinness. Vansteelandt el al. [37] explained high levels of physical activity in ED throughout psychological mechanisms and emphasized the fact that AN and BN patients have place too much value in their body shape and weight. Thus, physical activity is a result of a conscious attempt to work-off calories and obtain their desired thinness ideal, making the drive for thinness an important motive to engage in PPA. This is also the case in the general population, where weight and shape control reasons for exercise participation are very common [97].

4.5. Problematic Use of Physical Activity and Weight, BMI and Body Composition

Findings should be interpreted with caution due to the absence of validated methods to assess body composition in ED patients [98]. In both our classification and independently of ED types (AN and BN), almost half the studies did not find an association between different intensities of physical activity and BMI or body composition. The other half found a significantly positive association between PPA and body weight, BMI or percentage of body fat. It is in accordance with the findings of Bouten et al. [46] who showed that there was a threshold of BMI at 17 kg·m^{-2} among adult AN outpatients under which patients decreased their physical activity. They tried explaining these decreases in PPA and BMI with a decrease in muscle mass, diminished muscular function, malnutrition and exhaustion [46]. This goes in agreement with the findings of [39], who suggested that an increased physical activity occurs in AN patients during weight gain and recovery periods, as well as during the treatment phase and restoration of body fat [73].

4.6. Problematic Use of Physical Activity Link with Age of Onset, Age and Lifetime Activity Status in AN

Very few studies adjusted their results to age. In Group 1, only the larger study over two studies [61,67] found that PPA was associated with a younger age at time of interview but this was in a sample of ED where AN and BN patients where not distinguished [61]. Two explanations were proposed for this result: (1) the easy access to exercise behaviors as a weight-control mechanism at younger ages, rather than having access to other purging behaviors such as laxatives and purgatives; (2) the existence of an inverse relationship between exercise and age, which is also found in the general population, where physical activity tends to decrease with age [99].

In addition, PPA in Group 2 was related to physical activity during childhood: Davis et al. [48,50] found that AN patients who had been highly active as children were found to be engaged in more PPA during their illness. These findings suggest that high levels of physical activity during childhood could predict the development of PPA in AN, implying possible individual profile variations independently of the disorder. This goes in agreement with findings from the general population implying that sports participation during childhood and adolescence is particularly predictive of being more physically active later in life [99].

4.7. Problematic Use of Physical Activity and AN Treatment Outcome

The contradictory results between two studies [70,73] that, respectively, included adults and adolescents, raise the question of the contribution of age to the results. Indeed, there is a lower frequency of dropout in teens [100] combined with the lowest severity of ED at adolescence [101], and higher physical activity during childhood and adolescence than among young adults and older age groups [102].

4.8. Problematic Use of Physical Activity and Compulsivity

Continuing normal to high activity levels despite weight loss and a negative energy balance is recognized as an exclusive specificity of AN patients compared to individuals in a situation of starvation due to other causes such as those implicating an increase in circulating inflammatory cytokines [103] in humans as well in animal models [104,105].

In animal models mimicking several symptoms of AN in an attempt to give a rather biological approach, a reduction in food intake and body weight was paradoxically accompanied by a progressive increased activity level. The most described animal model combining food restriction and voluntary physical activity is the "Activity-Based Anorexia" model (ABA model) developed in the rat by Routtenberg and Kuznesof [106], then in the mouse. This model is also called "starvation-induced hyperactivity" [107] or "semi-starvation induced hyperactivity" [108]. In fact, the rodents have free access to a running wheel and showed hyperactivity occurring in response to a limited food supply due to limited access time to food (1–2 h per day). Such behavior, occurring at 2–3 days after the beginning of the protocol, led to feedback inhibition of food intake or self-starvation and death in 5–6 days [109]. Thus, the negative energy balance state that becomes life threatening, eventually leads to death [2,110]. A lot of research has been done on animal models to try understanding and determining the biological phenomenon underneath this particular hyperactivity, which occurred several hours before food distribution and is called food anticipatory activity. Similar activity has been also described in AN patients [111]. The animal models will not be detailed as it is beyond the scope of this systematic review.

4.9. A Proposed Comprehensive Model of the Development of PPA in AN

At this point, we can propose, based on literature reviews and clinical practice, a comprehensive model of the development of PPA in AN (Figure 2), taking into account both the history of the patient, his/her interaction with his/her environment and the pathological consequences of AN. This model is divided into five periods: Period 0 entitled "factors preceding AN", Period 1 entitled "onset of AN", Period 2 entitled "evolution of AN", Period 3 entitled "acute phase of AN" and Period 4 entitled "long-term outcome". In parallel, these periods evolve in three clinical phases (number 1, 2 and 3), with voluntary and involuntary components varying with time.

- In Period 0: The main points that should be taken into account are a patient's childhood activity profile [48], having a more physically active father [58], participation in esthetic- or weight-oriented sports [112]. An increase in PPA is observed one year prior to the onset of the disease [48].
- In Period 1: An increased PPA is majored with an early age of onset [61]; PPA as a conscious strategy for AN patients to optimize weight loss, also found in the general population [9,97].

Clinical phase number 1: Patients program a physical activity determined in defined moments of the day. This physical activity progressively increases in volume, intensity and/or frequency. PPA is described by patients as voluntary [10] and "goal-directed, organized and planned" [23].

- In Period 2: PPA becomes a coping strategy to compensate, suppress, and/or alleviate both negative affective states (anxiety [54,56], depression [54] and stress [20,75]) and ED symptoms [75] including, weight preoccupation [45,58], drive for thinness [40,51,74] body dissatisfaction [40] and restrictive profile [63,65].
- This is in addition modulated by ambient temperature [67].

Clinical phase number 2: As the ED progresses, physical activity could become an increasingly autonomous process. Involuntary PPA appears, with automation of the behavior. For example: patients run instead of walking, stand up when they normally should be sitting down, for example while writing or eating, or walk instead of standing still. This PPA is associated with diffuse restlessness and a significant unsteadiness, where the patient is literally unable to stand still for a short period. At a certain point, patients will even maintain muscular tension such as keeping their gluteal or abdominal muscles contracted without even thinking about it. The latter is called "static PPA". Furthermore, patients will continue to try to maximize their daily energy expenditure by all voluntary means possible. For example, they walk to get from one place to another instead of using a car, use stairs instead of elevators, do more housework, etc.

- In period 3: PPA has now a composite nature. It has a compulsive component not under voluntary cognitive control of the patient [9], irrespective of the antecedent motivation to exercise. Nevertheless, patients also present voluntary PPA due to a current context (for example: increased activity motivated by body dissatisfaction and weight preoccupation such as weight increase). The respective proportions of voluntary vs. involuntary PPA vary in a given subject both according to patients themselves and according to time. Clinical practice suggests, as it has been observed in biological animal models that a small subgroup of patients could (or can) be hyperactive until death with a huge hyperactivity despite very low weight.

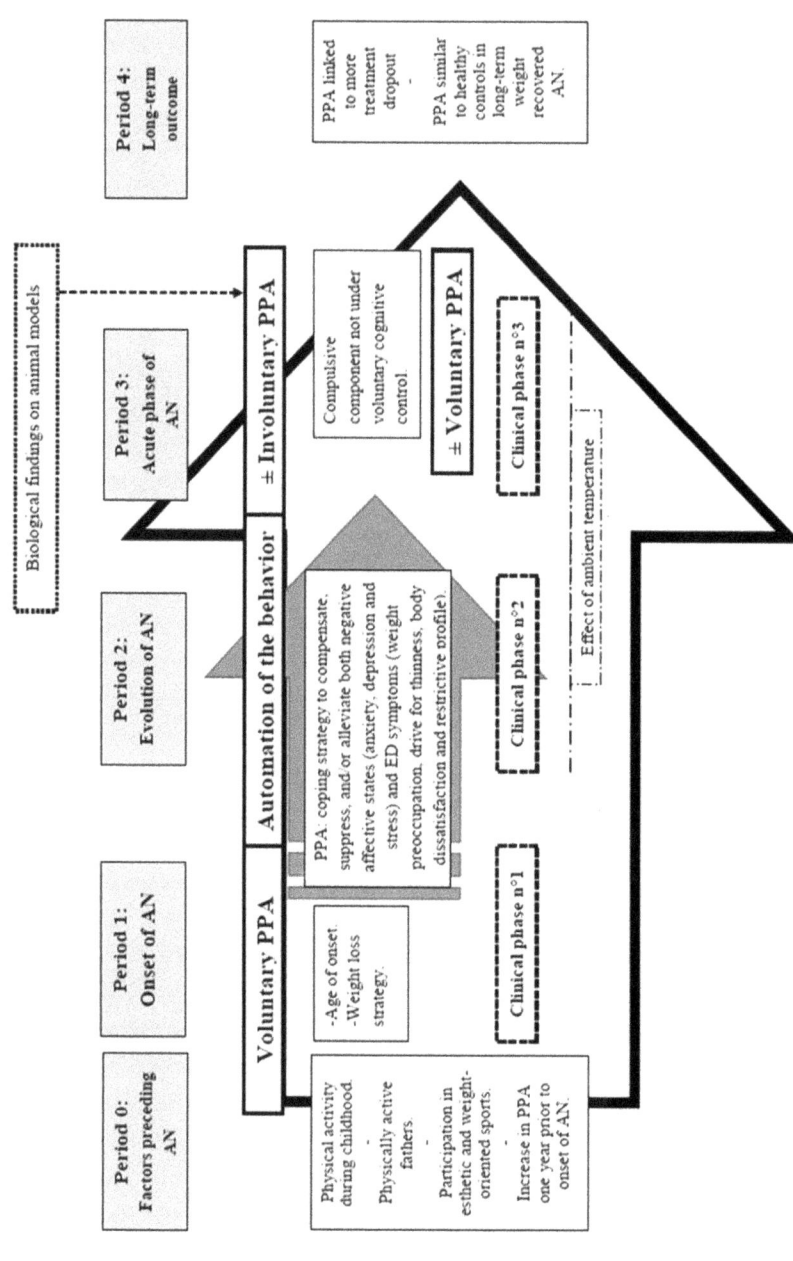

Figure 2. Proposed comprehensive model of development of problematic use of physical activity (PPA) in AN.

Clinical phase number 3: PPA is described by patients as "more intense, driven, disorganized and aimless than it was" [23] and as "aimless, stereotyped and inefficient" [10]. This phase associates clinical manifestations number 1 and 2, with varying degrees. We can notice here three profiles of patients: (1) hypo- or normal-active patients; (2) patients who relatively control important PPA; (3) patients who can't control their extremely important and solitary PPA (sometimes until death), associated unsteadiness and static physical activity.

– In period 4: A Long-term outcome is not very well known. Long-term weight recovered patients have been found to have a frequency of PPA similar to healthy controls [39]. Furthermore, PPA seemed to be associated with more dropout [70] and could be a negative factor for the extremely active patients.

4.10. Limitations

It is important to acknowledge the limitations of our work. Firstly, the term "problematic use of physical activity" is a term we have decided to use. Unfortunately, it does add to the plethora of terms already found in the litterature. This highlights the urgent need for the development of an international and interdisciplinary task force that would need to find and vote on a commonly accepted term and definition. Secondly, some studies [45,49,50,52,74,75,83] were added in both groups 1 and 2 because they evaluated PPA both quantitatively and qualitatively. Despite the fact that this had been taken into account while analysing the results of these specific studies, it can still be considered as an external bias. Finally, our model is an attemp to synthetise the elements of the literature, the clinical elements we collected from persons with AN, in order to better understand PPA. All individuals with AN do not have PPA or exactly the same PPA. The component we described can be present at the same time or at different times. We hope that this model will help explain the complexity of the phenomen and help treat it better.

5. Conclusions

Having no consensus definition for what is PPA in ED, the interpretation of previous studies findings can be partially jeopardized. In order to address this problem, we attempt to propose in our review a definition of this clinical concept including quantitative (intensity, frequency, duration and type of physical activity) and qualitative (motives for exercise, compulsiveness and exercise dependence/addiction) elements only in AN, given that very little information was found on BN. Thus, this paper highlights two main opposite component of PPA in AN: (a) PPA that is sometimes voluntarily increased in AN for the soul purpose of burning-off more calories and thus viewed as a conscious strategy of AN patients to optimize weight loss; (b) PPA that sometimes is involuntarily increased simultaneously with weight-loss and low ambient temperatures; indicating that exercise might not be under voluntary cognitive control of the patient, with a subconscious biological drive, a part of this activity becoming totally automatic. Additionally, according to the literature and clinical experience, a chronological model for the development of PPA in AN patient was proposed encompassing five periods evolving into three clinical stages.

In conclusion, we hypothesized that the evaluation of the intensity, frequency, duration and type of physical activity along with the motives for exercise, compulsiveness and exercise dependence for each person with ED would allow more individualized and efficient medical therapies.

Future research initiatives should focus on finding and voting on a commonly accepted term and definition for PPA in ED.

Author Contributions: Conceptualization, R.M. and G.N.; Methodology, R.M., M.L. and G.N.; Validation, K.L., B.S., D.J. and V.O.; Investigation, R.M., M.L., K.L. and G.N.; Data Curation, R.M., M.L. and G.N.; Writing—Original Draft Preparation, R.M., M.L. and G.N.; Writing—Review & Editing, R.M., M.L. and G.N.; Visualization, R.M. and G.N.; Supervision, G.N. All authors have read and agreed to the published version of the manuscript.

Funding: This research received no external funding.

Conflicts of Interest: The authors declare no conflict of interest.

References

1. Gull, W. Anorexia Nervosa. *Philos. Trans. R. Soc. Lond.* **1874**, *7*, 22–28. [CrossRef]
2. Hebebrand, J.; Exner, C.; Hebebrand, K.; Hotlkamk, C.; Casper, R.C.; Remschmidt, H.; Herpertz-Dahlmann, B.; Klingenspor, M. Hyperactivity in patients with anorexia nervosa and in semistarved rats: Evidence for a pivotal role of hypoleptinemia. *Physiol. Behav.* **2003**, *79*, 25–37. [CrossRef]
3. Solenberger, S. Exercise and eating disorders: A 3-years inpatient hospital record analysis. *Eat. Behav.* **2001**, *2*, 151–168. [CrossRef]
4. Taranis, L.T.; Meyer, C.M. Associations between specific components of compulsive exercise and eating-disordered cognitions and behaviors among young women. *Int. J. Eat. Disord.* **2011**, *44*, 452–458. [CrossRef]
5. Ng, L.; Ng, D.; Wong, W. Is supervised exercise training safe in patients with anorexia nervosa? A meta-analysis. *Physiotherapy* **2013**, *99*, 1–11. [CrossRef]
6. Strober, M.; Freeman, R.; Morrell, W. The long-term course of severe anorexia nervosa in adolescents: Survival analysis of recovery, relapse, and outcome predictors over 10–15 years in a prospective study. *Int. J. Eat. Disord.* **1997**, *22*, 339–360. [CrossRef]
7. Caspersen, C.J.; Powell, K.E.; Christenson, G.M. Physical activity, exercise & physical fitness: Definitions & Distinctions for Health-Related Research. *Public Health Rep.* **1985**, *100*, 126–131.
8. Hagger, M. Avoiding the "déjà variable" phenomenon: Social psychology needs more guides to constructs. *Front. Psychol.* **2014**, *5*, 52. [CrossRef]
9. Davis, C. Eating Disorders and Hyperactivity: A Psychobiological Perspective. *Can. J. Psychiatry* **1997**, *42*, 168–175. [CrossRef] [PubMed]
10. Kohl, M.; Foulon, C.; Guelfi, J.-D. Aspects comportementaux et biologiques de l'hyperactivité dans l'anorexie mentale. *L'Encephale* **2004**, *30*, 492–499. [CrossRef]
11. Meyer, C.; Taranis, L. Exercise in the Eating Disorders: Terms and Definitions. *Eur. Eat. Disord. Rev.* **2011**, *19*, 169–174. [CrossRef]
12. Meyer, C.; Taranis Goodwin, H.; Haycraft, E. Compulsive Exercise and Eating Disorders. *Eur. Eat. Disord. Rev.* **2011**, *19*, 174–189. [CrossRef] [PubMed]
13. Gümmer, R.; Giel, K.E.; Schag, K.; Resmark, G.; Junne, F.P.; Becker, S.; Zipfel, S.; Teufel, M. High Levels of Physical Activity in Anorexia Nervosa: A Systematic Review. *Eur. Eat. Disord. Rev.* **2015**, *23*, 333–344. [CrossRef] [PubMed]
14. Achamrah, N.; Nobis, S.; Breton, J.; Jésus, P.; Belmonte, L.; Maurer, B.; Coëffier, M.; Legrand, R.; Bôle-Feysot, C.; do Rego, J.L.; et al. Maintaining physical activity during refeeding improves body composition, intestinal hyperpermeability and behavior in anorectic mice. *Sci. Rep.* **2016**, *6*. [CrossRef] [PubMed]
15. Hagger, M. What makes a 'good' review article? Some reflections and recommendations. *Health Psychol. Rev.* **2012**, *6*, 141–146. [CrossRef]
16. Dishman, R.K. Medical psychology in exercise and sport. *Med. Clin. N. Am.* **1985**, *69*, 123–143. [CrossRef]
17. Adkins, E.; Keel, P. Does "Excessive" or "Compulsive" Best Describe Exercise as a Symptom of Bulimia Nervosa? *Int. J. Eat. Disord.* **2005**, *38*, 24–29. [CrossRef]
18. Moher, D.; Liberati, A.; Tetzlaff, J.; Altman, D.G. Preferred Reporting Items for Systematic Reviews and Meta-Analyses: The PRISMA Statement. *PLoS Med.* **2009**, *6*, 1–7. [CrossRef]
19. Blumenthal, J.A.; O'Toole, L.C.; Chang, J.L. Is running an analogue of anorexia nervosa? An empirical study of obligatory running and anorexia nervosa. *JAMA* **1984**, *252*, 520–523. [CrossRef]
20. Crisp, A.; Hsu, L.; Harding, B.; Hartshorn, J. Clinical features of anorexia nervosa: A study of a consecutive series of 102 female patients. *J. Psychosom. Res.* **1980**, *24*, 179–191. [CrossRef]
21. Davis, C.; Kennedy, S.H.; Ravelski, E.; Dionne, M. The role of physical activity in the development and maintenance of eating disorders. *Psychol. Med.* **1994**, *24*, 957–967.
22. Frey, J.; Hebebrand, J.; Müller, B.; Ziegler, A.; Blum, W.; Remschmidt, H.; Herpertz-Dahlmann, B. Reduced body fat in long-term followed-up female patients with anorexia nervosa. *J. Psychiatr. Res.* **2000**, *34*, 83–88. [CrossRef]

23. Kron, L.; Katz, J.; Gorzynski, G.; Weiner, H. Hyperactivity in Anorexia Nervosa: A Fundamental Clinical Feature. *Compr. Psychiatry* **1978**, *19*, 433–440. [CrossRef]

24. Monell, E.; Levallius, J.; Mantilla, E.; Birgegård, A. Running on empty—A nationwide large-scale examination of compulsive exercise in eating disorders. *J. Eat. Disord.* **2018**, *6*, 11. [CrossRef]

25. Sharp, C.; Clark, S.; Dunan, J.; Blackwood, D.; Shapiro, C. Clinical Presentation of Anorexia Nervosa in Males: 24 New Cases. *Int. J. Eat. Disord.* **1994**, *15*, 125–134. [CrossRef]

26. Higgins, J.; Hagman, J.; Zhaoxing, P.; MacLean, P. Increased Physical Activity Not Decreased Energy Intake Is Associated with Inpatient Medical Treatment for Anorexia Nervosa in Adolescent Females. *PLoS ONE* **2013**. [CrossRef]

27. Long, C.; Hollin, C. Assessment and management of eating disordered patients who over-exercise: A four-year follow-up of six single case studies. *J. Ment. Health.* **1995**, *4*, 309–316. [CrossRef]

28. Boyd, C.; Abraham, S.; Luscombe, G. Exercise Behaviours and Feelings in Eating Disorder and Non-Eating Disorder Groups. *Eur. Eat. Disord. Rev.* **2007**, *15*, 112–118. [CrossRef]

29. Bratland-Sanda, S.; Sundgot-Borgen, J.; Rø, Ø.; Rosenvinge, J.; Hoffart, A.; Martinsen, E. Physical Activity and Exercise Dependence during Inpatient Treatment of Longstanding Eating Disorders: An Exploratory Study of Excessive and Non-Excessive Exercisers. *Int. J. Eat. Disord.* **2010**, *43*, 266–273. [CrossRef]

30. Bratland-Sanda, S.; Sundgot-Borgen, J.; Rø, Ø.; Rosenvinge, J.; Hoffart, A.; Martinsen, E. "I'm Not Physically Active-I Only Go for Walks": Physical Activity in Patients with Longstanding Eating Disorders. *Int. J. Eat. Disord.* **2010**, *43*, 88–92. [CrossRef]

31. Bratland-Sanda, S.; Martinsen, E.; Rosenvinge, J.; Rø, Ø.; Hoffart, A.; Sundgot-Borgen, J. Exercise Dependence Score in Patients with Longstanding Eating Disorders and Controls: The Importance of Affect Regulation and Physical Activity Intensity. *Eur. Eat. Disord. Rev.* **2011**, *19*, 249–255. [CrossRef] [PubMed]

32. Carruth, B.; Skinner, J. Bone Mineral Status in Adolescent Girls: Effects of Eating Disorders and Exercise. *J. Adolesc. Health* **2000**, *26*, 322–329. [CrossRef]

33. Davis, C.; Kaptein, S.; Kaplan, A.; Olmsted, M.; Woodside, B. Obsessionality in Anorexia Nervosa: The Moderating Influence of Exercise. *Psychosom. Med.* **1998**, *60*, 192–197. [CrossRef] [PubMed]

34. Hechler, T.; Rieger, E.; Touyz, S.; Beumont, P. Physical Activity and Body Composition in Outpatients Recovering from Anorexia Nervosa and Healthy Controls. *Adapt. Phys. Activ. Q.* **2008**, *25*, 159–173. [CrossRef]

35. Naylor, N.; Mountford, V.; Brown, G. Beliefs about Excessive Exercise in Eating Disorders: The Role of Obsessions and Compulsions. *Eur. Eat. Disord. Rev.* **2011**, *19*, 226–236. [CrossRef]

36. Stiles-Shields, C.; Goldschmidt, A.; Boepple, L.; Glunz, C.; Le Grange, D. Driven Exercise Among Treatment-Seeking Youth with Eating disorders. *Eat. Behav.* **2011**, *12*, 328–331. [CrossRef]

37. Vansteelandt, K.; Rijmen, F.; Pieters, G.; Probst, M.; Vanderlinden, J. Drive for thinness, affect regulation and physical activity in eating disorders: A daily life study. *Behav. Res. Ther.* **2007**, *45*, 1717–1734. [CrossRef]

38. Falk, J.; Halmi, K.; Tryon, W. Activity measures in anorexia nervosa. *Arch. Gen. Psychiatry* **1985**, *42*, 811–814. [CrossRef]

39. Kaye, W.; Gwirtsman, H.; George, T.; Ebert, M.; Petersen, R. Caloric Consumption and Activity Levels After Weight Recovery in Anorexia Nervosa: A Prolonged Delay in Normalization. *Int. J. Eat. Disord.* **1986**, *5*, 489–502. [CrossRef]

40. Casper, R.; Schoeller, D.; Kushner, R.; Hnilicka, J.; Trainer Gold, S. Total daily energy expenditure and activity level in anorexia nervosa. *Am. J. Clin. Nutr.* **1991**, *53*, 1143–1150. [CrossRef]

41. Pirke, K.; Trimborn, P.; Platte, P.; Fichter, M. Average Total Energy Expenditure in Anorexia Nervosa, Bulimia Nervosa, and Healthy Young Women. *Biol. Psychiatry* **1991**, *30*, 711–718. [CrossRef]

42. Long, C.G.; Smith, J.; Midgley, M.; Cassidy, T. Over-exercising in anorexic and normal samples: Behaviour and attitudes. *J. Ment. Health* **1993**, *2*, 321–327. [CrossRef]

43. Carmack, M.A.; Martins, R. Measuring commitment to running: A survey of runners' attitudes and mental states. *J. Sport Exerc. Psychol.* **1979**, *1*, 25–42. [CrossRef]

44. Brewerton, T.; Stellefson, E.; Hibbs, N.; Hodges, E.; Cochrane, C. Comparison of Eating Disorder Patients with and Without Compulsive Exercising. *Int. J. Eat. Disord.* **1995**, *17*, 413–416. [CrossRef]

45. Davis, C.; Kennedy, S.; Ralevski, E.; Dionne, M.; Brewer, H.; Neitzert, C.; Ratusny, D. Obsessive compulsiveness and physical activity in anorexia nervosa and high-level exercising. *J. Psychosom. Res.* **1995**, *39*, 967–976. [CrossRef]

46. Bouten, C.; Van Marken Lichtenbelt, W.; Westerterp, K. Body Mass Index and daily physical activity in Anorexia Nervosa. *Med. Sci. Sports Exerc.* **1996**, *28*, 967–973. [CrossRef]

47. Casper, R.; Jabine, L. An Eight-Year Follow-Up: Outcome from Adolescent Compared to Adult Onset Anorexia Nervosa. *J. Youth Adolesc.* **1996**, *25*, 499–517. [CrossRef]

48. Davis, C.; Katzman, D.K.; Kaptein, S.; Kirsh, C.; Brewer, H.; Kalmbach, K.; Olmsted, M.F.; Woodside, D.B.; Kaplan, A.S. The Prevalence of High-Level Exercise in the Eating Disorders: Etiological Implications. *Compr. Psychiatry* **1997**, *38*, 321–326. [CrossRef]

49. Davis, C.; Claridge, G. The eating disorders as addiction: A psychobiological perspective. *Addict. Behav.* **1998**, *23*, 463–475. [CrossRef]

50. Davis, C.; Katzman, D.; Kirsh, C. Compulsive Physical Activity in Adolescents with Anorexia Nervosa: A Psychobehavioral Spiral of Pathology. *J. Nerv. Ment. Dis.* **1999**, *187*, 336–342. [CrossRef]

51. Favaro, A.; Caregaro, L.; Burlina, A.; Santonastaso, P. Tryptophan Levels, Excessive Exercise, and Nutritional Status in Anorexia Nervosa. *Psychosom. Med.* **2000**, *62*, 535–538. [CrossRef] [PubMed]

52. Pinkston, M.; Martz, D.; Domer, F.; Curtin, L.; Bazzini, D.; Smith, L.; Henson, D. Psychological, nutritional & energy expenditure in college females with Anorexia Nervosa vs. comparable-mass control. *Eat. Behav.* **2001**, *2*, 169–181. [PubMed]

53. Davis, C.; Woodside, B. Sensitivity to the Rewarding Effects of Food and Exercise in the Eating Disorders. *Compr. Psychiatry* **2002**, *43*, 189–194. [CrossRef] [PubMed]

54. Penas-Lledo, E.; Vaz Leal, F.; Waller, G. Excessive exercise in anorexia nervosa & boulimia nervosa: Relations to eating characteristics & general psychopathology. *Int. J. Eat. Disord.* **2002**, *31*, 370–375. [PubMed]

55. Holtkamp, K.; Herpertz-Dahlmann, B.; Mika, C.; Heer, M.; Heussen, N.; Fichter, M.; Herpertz, S.; Senf, W.; Blum, W.; Schweiger, U.; et al. Elevated Physical Activity and Low Leptin Levels Co-occur in Patients with Anorexia Nervosa. *J. Clin. Endocrinol. Metab.* **2003**, *88*, 5169–5174. [CrossRef] [PubMed]

56. Holtkamp, K.; Hebebrand, J.; Herpertz-Dahlmann, B. The Contribution of Anxiety and Food Restriction on Physical Activity Levels in Acute Anorexia Nervosa. *Int. J. Eat. Disord.* **2004**, *36*, 163–171. [CrossRef] [PubMed]

57. Klein, D.; Bennett, A.; Schebendach, J.; Foltin, R.; Devlin, M.; Walsh, T. Exercise "Addiction" in Anorexia Nervosa: Model Development and Pilot Data. *CNS Spectr.* **2004**, *9*, 531–537. [CrossRef]

58. Davis, C.; Blackmore, E.; Katzman, D.K.; Fox, J. Female adolescents with anorexia nervosa and their parents: A case-control study of exercise attitudes and behaviours. *Psychol. Med.* **2005**, *35*, 377–386. [CrossRef]

59. Davis, C.; Kaptein, S. Anorexia nervosa with excessive exercise: A phenotype with close links to obsessive-compulsive disorder. *Psychiatry Res.* **2006**, *142*, 209–217. [CrossRef]

60. Holtkamp, K.; Herpertz-Dahlmann, B.; Hebebrand, K.; Mika, C.; Kratzsch, J.; Hebebrand, J. Physical Activity and Restlessness Correlate with Leptin Levels in Patients with Adolescent Anorexia Nervosa. *Biol. Psychiatry* **2006**, *60*, 311–313. [CrossRef]

61. Shroff, H.; Reba, L.; Thornton, L.; Tozzi, F.; Klump, K.; Berrettini, W.; Brandt, H.; Crawford, S.; Crow, S.; Fichter, M.; et al. Features Associated with Excessive Exercise in Women with Eating Disorders. *Int. J. Eat. Disord.* **2006**, *39*, 454–461. [CrossRef] [PubMed]

62. Klein, D.; Mayer, L.; Schebendach, J.; Walsh, T. Physical activity and cortisol in Anorexia Nervosa. *Psychoneuroendocrinology* **2007**, *32*, 539–547. [CrossRef] [PubMed]

63. Dalle Grave, R.; Calugi, S.; Marchesini, G. Compulsive exercise to control shape or weight in eating disorders: Prevalence, associated features, and treatment outcome. *Compr. Psychiatry* **2008**, *49*, 346–352. [CrossRef] [PubMed]

64. Mond, J.; Calogero, R. Excessive exercise in eating disorder patients and in healthy women. *Aust. N. Z. J. Psychiatry* **2009**, *43*, 227–234. [CrossRef]

65. Bewell-Weiss, C.; Carter, J. Predictors of excessive exercise in anorexia nervosa. *Compr. Psychiatry* **2010**, *51*, 566–571. [CrossRef]

66. Thornton, L.; Dellava, J.; Root, T.; Lichtenstein, P.; Bulik, C. Anorexia nervosa and generalized anxiety disorder: Further explorations of the relation between anxiety and body mass index. *J. Anxiety Disord.* **2011**, *25*, 727–730. [CrossRef]

67. Carrera, O.; Adan, R.; Gutierrez, E.; Danner, U.; Hoek, H.; Elburg, A.; Kas, M. Hyperactivity in Anorexia Nervosa: Warming Up Not Just Burning-Off Calories. *PLoS ONE* **2012**, *7*, e41851. [CrossRef]

68. Murray, S.; Rieger, E.; Hildebrandt, T.; Karlov, L.; Russel, J.; Boon, E.; Dawson, R.; Touyz, S. A comparison of eating, exercise, shape, and weight related symptomatology in males with muscle dysmorphia and anorexia nervosa. *Body Image* **2012**, *9*, 193–200. [CrossRef]

69. Smith, A.; Fink, E.; Anestis, M.; Ribeiro, J.; Gordon, K.; Davis, H.; Keel, P.; Bardone-Cone, A.; Peterson, C.; Klein, M.; et al. Exercise caution: Over-exercise is associated with suicidality among individuals with disordered eating. *Psychiatry Res.* **2012**, *206*, 246–255. [CrossRef]

70. El Ghoch, M.; Calugi, S.; Pellegrini, M.; Milanese, C.; Busacchi, M.; Battistini, N.C.; Bernabe, J.; Dalle Grave, R. Measured Physical Activity in Anorexia Nervosa: Features and Treatment Outcome. *Int. J. Eat. Disord.* **2013**. [CrossRef]

71. Alberti, M.; Galvani, C.; El Ghoch, M.; Capelli, C.; Lanza, M.; Calugi, S.; Dalle Grave, R. Assessment of Physical Activity in Anorexia Nervosa and Treatment Outcome. *Med. Sci. Sports Exerc.* **2013**, *45*, 1643–1648. [CrossRef]

72. Brownstone, L.; Fitzsimmons-Craft, E.; Wonderlich, S.; Joiner, T.; Le Grange, D.; Mitchell, J.; Crow, S.J.; Peterson, C.B.; Crosby, R.D.; Klein, M.H.; et al. Hard exercise, affect lability, and personality among individuals with bulimia nervosa. *Eat. Behav.* **2013**, *14*, 413–419. [CrossRef] [PubMed]

73. Kostrzewa, E.; van Elburg, A.; Sanders, N.; Sternheim, L.; Adan, R.; Kas, M. Longitudinal Changes in the Physical Activity of Adolescents with Anorexia Nervosa and Their Influence on Body Composition and Leptin Serum Levels after Recovery. *PLoS ONE* **2013**, *8*, e78251. [CrossRef] [PubMed]

74. Zipfel, S.; Mack, I.; Baur, L.A.; Hebebrand, J.; Touyz, S.; Herzog, W.; Abraham, S.; Davies, P.S.; Russell, J. Impact of exercise on energy metabolism in anorexia nervosa. *J. Eat. Disord.* **2013**, *1*, 37. [CrossRef] [PubMed]

75. Keyes, A.; Woerwag-Mehta, S.; Bartholdy, S.; Koskina, A.; Middleton, B.; Connan, F.; Webster, P.; Schmidt, U. Physical activity and the drive to exercise in anorexia nervosa. *Int. J. Eat. Disord.* **2015**, *48*, 46–54. [CrossRef] [PubMed]

76. Sauchelli, S.; Arcelus, J.; Sánchez, I.; Riesco, N.; Jiménez-Murcia, S.; Granero, R.; Gunnard, K.; Baños, R.; Botella, C.; Fernández-García, J.C.; et al. Physical activity in anorexia nervosa: How relevant is it to therapy response? *Eur. Psychiatry* **2015**, *30*, 924–931. [CrossRef] [PubMed]

77. Sternheim, L.; Danner, U.; Adan, R.; van Elburg, A. Drive for activity in patients with anorexia nervosa. *Int. J. Eat. Disord.* **2015**, *48*, 42–45. [CrossRef]

78. Blachno, M.; Brynska, A.; Tomaszewicz-Libudzic, C.; Jagielska, G.; Srebnicki, T.; Wisniewski, A.; Wolanczyk, T. Obsessive-compulsive symptoms and physical activity in patients with anorexia nervosa–possible relationships. *Psychiatr. Pol.* **2016**, *50*, 55–64. [CrossRef]

79. El Ghoch, M.; Calugi, S.; Pellegrini, M.; Chignola, E.; Dalle Grave, R. Physical activity, body weight, and resumption of menses in anorexia nervosa. *Psychiatry Res.* **2016**, *246*, 507–511. [CrossRef]

80. Gianini, L.M.; Klein, D.A.; Call, C.; Walsh, B.T.; Wang, Y.; Wu, P.; Attia, E. Physical activity and post-treatment weight trajectory in anorexia nervosa. *Int. J. Eat. Disord.* **2016**, *49*, 482–489. [CrossRef]

81. Noetel, M.; Miskovic-Wheatley, J.; Crosby, R.D.; Hay, P.; Madden, S.; Touyz, S. A clinical profile of compulsive exercise in adolescent inpatients with anorexia nervosa. *J. Eat. Disord.* **2016**, *4*, 1. [CrossRef] [PubMed]

82. Lehmann, C.; Hofmann, T.; Elbelt, U.; Rose, M.; Correll, C.; Stengel, A.; Haas, V. The Role of Objectively Measured, Altered Physical Activity Patterns for Body Mass Index Change during Inpatient Treatment in Female Patients with Anorexia Nervosa. *J. Clin. Med.* **2018**, *7*, 289. [CrossRef] [PubMed]

83. Schlegl, S.; Dittmer, N.; Hoffmann, S.; Voderholzer, U. Self-reported quantity compulsiveness and motives of exercise in patients with eating disorders and healthy controls: Differences and similarities. *J. Eat. Disord.* **2018**, *6*, 17. [CrossRef] [PubMed]

84. Young, S.; Touyz, S.; Meyer, C.; Arcelus, J.; Rhodes, P.; Madden, S.; Pike, K.; Attia, E.; Crosby, R.O.; Hay, P. Relationships between compulsive exercise, quality of life, psychological distress and motivation to change in adults with anorexia nervosa. *J. Eat. Disord.* **2018**, *6*, 2. [CrossRef] [PubMed]

85. Ainsworth, B.; Haskell, W.; Whitt, M.; Irwin, M.; Swartz, A.; Strath, S.; O'Brien, W.; Bassett, D.; Schmitz, K.; Emplaincourt, P.; et al. Compendium of Physical Activities: An update of activity codes and MET intensities. *Med. Sci. Sports Exerc.* **2000**, *32*, S498–S516. [CrossRef]

86. Lazare, A.; Klerman, G.L.; Armour, D.J. Oral obsessive and hysterical personality patterns: An investigation of psychoanalytic concepts by means of factor analysis. *JAMA Psychiatry* **1966**, *14*, 624–630. [CrossRef]

87. Lazare, A.; Klerman, G.L.; Armour, D.J. Oral, obsessive and hysterical personality patterns. Replication of factor analysis in an independent sample. *J. Psychiatr. Res.* **1970**, *7*, 275–290. [CrossRef]

88. Van Oppen, P.; Hoekstra, R.J.; Emmelkamp, P.M.G. The structure of obsessive-compulsive symptoms. *Behav. Res. Ther.* **1995**, *33*, 15–23. [CrossRef]
89. Mattar, L.; Godart, N.; Melchior, J.-C.; Falissard, B.; Kolta, S.; Ringuenet, D.; Vindreau, C.; Nordon, C.; Blanchet, C.; Pichard, C. Underweight patients with anorexia nervosa: Comparison of bioelectrical impedance analysis using five equations to dual X-ray absorptiometry. *Clin. Nutr.* **2011**, *30*, 746–752. [CrossRef]
90. Cook, B.; Engel, S.; Crosby, R.; Hausenblas, H.; Wonderlich, S.; Mitchell, J. Pathological Motivations for Exercise and Eating Disorder Specific Health-Related Quality of Life. *Int. J. Eat. Disord.* **2014**, *47*, 268–272. [CrossRef]
91. Bezzina, L.; Touyz, S.; Young, S.; Foroughi, N.; Clemes, S.; Meyer, C.; Arcelus, J.; Madden, S.; Attia, E.; Hay, P.; et al. Accuracy of self-reported physical activity in patients with anorexia nervosa: Links with clinical features. *J. Eat. Disord.* **2019**, *7*, 28. [CrossRef]
92. Casper, R. Behavioral activation and lack of concern, core symptoms of anorexia nervosa. *Int. J. Eat. Disord.* **1998**, *24*, 381–393. [CrossRef]
93. Godart, N.; Flament, M.; Perdereau, F.; Jeammet, P. Comorbidity between eating disorders and anxiety disorders: A review. *Int. J. Eat. Disord.* **2002**, *32*, 253–270. [CrossRef]
94. Godart, N.; Perdereau, F.; Rein, Z.; Berthoz, S.; Wallier, J.; Jeammet, P.; Flament, M. Comorbidity studies of eating disorders and mood disorders. Critical review of the literature. *J. Affect. Disord.* **2007**, *97*, 37–49. [CrossRef] [PubMed]
95. Byrne, A.; Byrne, D. The effect of exercise on depression, anxiety, and other mood states: A Review. *J. Psychosom. Res.* **1993**, *37*, 565–574. [CrossRef]
96. Dunn, A.; Trivedi, M.; O'Neal, H. Physical activity dose-response effects on outcomes of depression and anxiety. *Med. Sci. Sports Exerc.* **2001**, *33*, S587–S597. [CrossRef] [PubMed]
97. Gonçalves, S.F.; Gomes, A.R. Exercising for weight and shape reasons vs. health control reasons: The impact on eating disturbance and psychological functioning. *Eat. Behav.* **2012**, *13*, 127–130. [CrossRef]
98. Mattar, L.; Godart, N.; Melchior, J.-C.; Pichard, C. Anorexia nervosa and nutritional assessment: Contribution of body composition measurements. *Nutr. Res. Rev.* **2011**, 1–7. [CrossRef]
99. Wall, M.; Carlson, S.; Stein, A.; Lee, S.; Fulton, J. Trends by Age in Youth Physical Activity: Youth Media Campaign Longitudinal Survey. *Med. Sci. Sports Exerc.* **2011**, *43*, 2140–2147. [CrossRef]
100. Wallier, J.; Vibert, S.; Berthoz, S.; Huas, C.; Hubert, T.; Godart, N. Dropout from Inpatient Treatment for Anorexia Nervosa: Critical Review of the Literature. *Int. J. Eat. Disord.* **2009**, *42*, 636–647. [CrossRef]
101. Hoang, U.; Goldacre, M.; James, A. Mortality following hospital discharge with a diagnosis of eating disorder: National record linkage study, England 2001–2009. *Int. J. Eat. Disord.* **2014**, *47*, 507–515. [CrossRef] [PubMed]
102. Owen, N.; Leslie, E.; Salmon, J.; Fotheringham, M. Environmental Determinants of Physical Activity and Sedentary Behavior. *Exerc. Sport Sci. Rev.* **2000**, *28*, 153–158. [PubMed]
103. Braun, T.; Marks, D. Pathophysiology and treatment of inflammatory anorexia in chronic disease. *J. Cachexia Sarcopenia Muscle* **2010**, *1*, 135–145. [CrossRef]
104. Baltgalvis, K.A.; Berger, F.G.; Peña, M.M.; Mark Davis, J.; White, J.P.; Carson, J.A. Activity level, apoptosis, and development of cachexia in Apc(Min/+) mice. *J. Appl. Physiol.* **2010**, *109*, 1155–1161. [CrossRef] [PubMed]
105. MacDonald, L.; Radler, M.; Paolini, A.G.; Kent, S. Calorie restriction attenuates LPS-induced sickness behavior and shifts hypothalamic signaling pathways to an anti-inflammatory bias. *Am. J. Physiol. Regul. Integr. Comp. Physiol.* **2011**, *301*, R172–R184. [CrossRef]
106. Routtenberg, A.; Kuznesof, A.W. Self-starvation of rats living in activity wheels on a restricted feeding schedule. *J. Comp. Physiol. Psychol.* **1967**, *64*, 414–421. [CrossRef]
107. Pirke, K.M.; Broocks, A.; Wilckens, T.; Marquard, R.; Schweiger, U. Starvation-induced hyperactivity in the rat: The role of endocrine and neurotransmitter changes. *Neurosci. Biobehav. Rev.* **1993**, *17*, 287–294. [CrossRef]
108. Exner, C.; Hebebrand, J.; Remschmidt, H.; Wewetzer, C.; Ziegler, A.; Herpertz, S.; Schweiger, U.; Blum, W.F.; Preibisch, G.; Heldmaier, G.; et al. Leptin suppresses semi-starvation induced hyperactivity in rats: Implications for anorexia nervosa. *Mol. Psychiatry* **2000**, *5*, 476–481. [CrossRef]
109. Adan, R.A.; Hillebrand, J.J.; Danner, U.N.; Cardona, S.; Kas, M.J.; Verhagen, L.A. Neurobiology driving hyperactivity in activity-based anorexia. *Curr. Top. Behav. Neurosci.* **2011**, *6*, 229–250.

110. Spatz, C.; Jones, S.D. Starvation anorexia as an explanation of "self-starvation" of rats living in activity wheels. *J. Comp. Physiol. Psychol.* **1971**, *77*, 313–317. [CrossRef]
111. Scheurink, A.; Boersma, G.; Nergardh, R.; Södersten, P. Neurobiology of hyperactivity and reward: Agreeable restlessness in Anorexia Nervosa. *Physiol. Behav.* **2010**, *100*, 490–495. [CrossRef] [PubMed]
112. Mitchison, D.; Hay, P. The epidemiology of eating disorders: Genetic, environmental, and societal factors. *Clin. Epidemiol.* **2014**, *17*, 89–97.

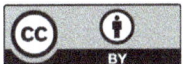

MDPI

St. Alban-Anlage 66

4052 Basel

Switzerland

Tel. +41 61 683 77 34

Fax +41 61 302 89 18

www.mdpi.com

Nutrients Editorial Office

E-mail: nutrients@mdpi.com

www.mdpi.com/journal/nutrients

www.ingramcontent.com/pod-product-compliance
Lightning Source LLC
Chambersburg PA
CBHW042022080526
44654CB00092B/223